The Breast Cancer Companion

A Guide for the Newly Diagnosed

The Breast Cancer Companion

A Guide for the Newly Diagnosed

Nancy Sokolowski, RN, OCN

Valerie Rossi

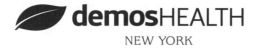

demosHEALTH

NEW YORK

Acquisitions Editor: Noreen Henson
Cover Design: Aimee Davis
Compositor: Absolute Service, Inc.
Printer: Hamilton Printing

Visit our Web site at www.demosmedpub.com

Library of Congress Cataloging-in-Publication Data

Sokolowski, Nancy.
   The breast cancer companion : a guide for the newly diagnosed / Nancy Sokolowski, Valerie Rossi.
      p. cm.
   Includes bibliographical references and index.
   ISBN 978-1-932603-99-6 (alk. paper)
   1.   Breast—Cancer—Popular works.   I. Rossi, Valerie. II. Title.
   RC280.B8S5854 2011
   616.99'449—dc22

                              2010021184

Special discounts on bulk quantities of Demos Health books are available to corporations, professional associations, pharmaceutical companies, healthcare organizations, and other qualifying groups. For details, please contact:

Special Sales Department
Demos Medical Publishing
11 W. 42nd Street
New York, NY 10036
Phone: 800–532–8663 or 212–683–0072
Fax: 212–941–7842
E-mail: rsantana@demosmedpub.com

Made in the United States of America
10 11 12 13   5 4 3 2 1

Contents

My Team and My Plans 57

Record Keeping 107

Resources 139

Foreword

Nationally recognized as an expert in the treatment of breast cancer, Dr. Richard Zelkowitz, or Dr. Z as he is affectionately called by his patients, is the medical director for the Smilow Family Breast Health Center and former chief of hematology and oncology at Norwalk Hospital.

The diagnosis—breast cancer—creates a feeling of crisis. You likely will be shocked. Your outlook on your health, your life, and your future may be shaken. This is all very normal.

How did this happen? The cause of breast cancer is mostly unknown. That does not help to know except to remove any possible guilty feelings you might have regarding your role in causing this cancer. The two major risk factors known are being a woman and getting older, and you have NO control over either. This loss of control introduces uncertainty. As time goes on, however, what will evolve out of uncertainty is personal growth, resilience, and strength as your priorities become clearer.

People often ask me how to choose the best medical team. You are about to enter a collaborative relationship with all members of the team that will be treating you. Most decisions will be made in conjunction with your doctors. Know that there is often more than one alternative that is appropriate for a given patient. For instance, you will be offered surgical options once the biopsy results are known. There are usually at least two choices—a lumpectomy followed by radiation or a mastectomy with or without breast reconstruction. The cure rate is the same for either.

Many factors will be considered in making this choice as well as the multitude of other decisions that will need to be made. Take your time. Gather all the data needed. Information from your medical team, Internet searches, books, organizations, friends, and family should be incorporated into your decision-making process. Once you have done that, your decisions will seem far easier. Trust your intuition; you will make the right choice.

Your relationship with your doctors is vital to your healing process. Although you need to be your own personal advocate, it is essential that a successful doctor–patient relationship be built on trust and communication. You must be comfortable sharing your fears and, more importantly, your questions with the doctors caring for you. This is not an area of compromise.

Patients also need some venue to air their concerns, whether that expression occurs with a doctor, nurse, other patient, or family and friends who are supportive. Writing in a journal, creative expression through art therapy or music therapy, or spiritual support can help with the evolution of your journey through this experience.

Physical and emotional healing is necessary for a complete recovery. Connecting with the correct healthcare team can offer enormous assistance with both. Knowledge provides some semblance of control when it appears there is none. Without concrete information, imaginations can be overactive causing fears that are unfounded.

As I read through this book for the first time, I could not help but think of my own personal journey with breast cancer. While I was in medical school, my mom was diagnosed with breast cancer. A woman who was my personal hero became ill in the prime of her life. I remember as she struggled with her fears and with the decisions she had to make. This was at a time when information was not nearly as accessible and when people certainly did not talk freely about such taboo topics such as cancer.

Over the years, I have had the honor of many women allowing me to share in their struggles as they embarked on their personal journey with breast cancer. We have come a long way medically since my mom was diagnosed, but we have an eternity yet to go.

I have also been fortunate for the last 20 years to have worked side by side with Nancy Sokolowski who shares my passion in meeting the needs confronting those stricken with breast cancer. Together we founded the Smilow Family Breast Health Center. She brings a positive attitude and tremendous energy to the caring and treatment of those who are fortunate enough to embrace her skills. She incorporated a vision of seamless care and services for women, their physicians, and the community. She has an amazing gift to relate to the multiple issues confronting women at this critical time. Through this timely book, Nancy's vast clinical and personal experience can now be shared. It is gratifying that her knowledge will continue to guide, inspire, and empower women newly diagnosed with breast cancer.

I wish you luck and success!

Richard Zelkowitz, MD
Medical Director
Smilow Family Breast Health Center

Introduction

It is our greatest hope that this book will provide guidance, organization, and timely "insider" tips to help your breast cancer treatment and recovery go as smoothly and successfully as it possibly can. We have compiled the best-of-the-best advice from the latest available research, from leading doctors in this field, from breast cancer survivors themselves, and from Nancy's 30 years of experience as one of the country's most respected and sought after breast healthcare specialist.

Val, herself coauthor of an award winning health organizer for people with type 2 diabetes, watched several friends go through the confusing and often overwhelming treatment and aftercare experiences that accompany a breast cancer diagnosis. She decided to use her publishing skills to help create a definitive, user-friendly guide to help women deal with the "what now" of that diagnosis. To do this, Val sought to collaborate with someone who was an expert in the full continuum of a women's treatment experience, from diagnosis to recovery. That search led her to Nancy. *The Breast Cancer Companion* is the result of that collaboration.

Nancy Sokolowski is uniquely positioned to coauthor *The Breast Cancer Companion*, having dedicated her extensive nursing career to women's medical issues. As cofounder of Norwalk Hospital's Smilow Family Breast Health Center, Nancy created a patient education center that focused on all aspects of breast healthcare services, including medical oncology, surgery, radiation oncology, pathology, breast and cervical early detection, and Wise Women screening programs.

Nancy also pioneered the role of the breast health navigator for newly diagnosed breast cancer patients, helping women find their way through myriad hospital services. She was responsible for a patient caseload of up to 250 women per year, advising them from diagnosis through to recovery. Nancy has been recognized on the national, state, and local levels as a leader in the physical and emotional care of women newly diagnosed with breast cancer. Her intense collaboration with Val on *The Breast Cancer Companion* is her way of sharing her vast storehouse of knowledge, process, and optimism with all women who have heard the words, "You have cancer."

We strongly feel that this book will greatly help you in your efforts to mount a smart, aggressive, organized, and ultimately successful battle with breast cancer. However, at the same time, we know that those efforts do not end with the last page of this book. In fact, we hope that you will keep this "companion" in plain view somewhere in your home as a gentle reminder to stay vigilant through every stage of your aftercare program.

For many, a cancer diagnosis is a catalyst for seeing and living life with more passion, and for some, reordering life's priorities. We hope that you experience this awakening, as many before you have, and that you come away actually strengthened by the journey that lies ahead! Live well to stay well!

Our best wishes,

Nancy Sokolowski and Val Rossi

Acknowledgments

The authors would like to express their heartfelt gratitude to the following.

To our amazing breast cancer survivors who generously gave of their time to read through our manuscripts and offer brilliant insights, suggestions, and inspirations for our readers: Ann Altchek, Cathy Colgan, Karen Como, Lynn Duchan, Claudia Francoeur, Gail Johnson, Shelly Kassen, Elizabeth Lewis, Eileen Margherio, Eileen Phelps, Linda Ruberto, Sue Ryan, Cathy Sutton, Catherine Stone, and Mary Taylor.

To Dr. Deanna DelPrete, for encouraging this project and for putting Nancy's business card in Val's hand.

To Janet Rosen, our literary agent, who believed in us and our book proposal and connected us with our publisher, Demos Health. We are especially grateful to have the passion and vision of our editor Noreen Henson and the staff of Demos Medical Publishing for expertly shepherding our manuscript to publication. We profusely thank Carlos Maldonado for his striking interior design and transforming our words, charts, and checklists into elegant and functional pages.

A special thanks to Dr. Richard Zelkowitz for being our guiding light, for his tireless devotion to the well-being of the breast cancer patient, and for exemplifying the best in extraordinary doctor–patient relationships. Your passion in meeting the extended needs of the individual inspires hope and has provided comfort for so many.

To Sara Rossi for painstakingly illustrating the prototype versions to give us a glimmer of what this book could be.

We would like to thank our families for encouraging and supporting our efforts at every turn, especially our husbands Todd Kolb and Dom Rossi, our most enthusiastic supporters.

How to Make This Book Work For You

The Breast Cancer Companion was created to help you feel organized and prepared at a time when so much feels uncertain and out of control. This book will help you organize your information so that your dates, contacts, questions, and notes will be at your fingertips throughout your treatments.

IN THE BEGINNING

To help you get started, read the chapter, **First Steps**. Here you will get a step-by-step guide of how to proceed after the initial diagnosis. You will find practical suggestions for gathering the information you need to be organized, informed, and ready for the consultations, tests, and decisions ahead of you.

To help with the countless forms that you will soon face, this planner has a place for you to fill in your health history, insurance information, and current medications. You can store names and numbers of your doctors and nurses, as well as your appointment dates in the **My Team and My Plans** chapter.

AT HOME

Use the **Journal and Appointments Notes** in this book for jotting down questions for your doctor, noting your symptoms and to do's, and planning your appointments and tests.

TREATMENTS

This book has checklists and tips to give you the peace of mind that you have thought of everything to be ready for your surgery, radiation, and/or chemotherapy treatments.

DOCTOR'S APPOINTMENTS

Bring this book to every doctor's appointment. **Review your Journal and Appointments Notes** for questions and symptoms that you would like to discuss with your doctor. The **Journal and Appointments Notes** is a good place to write down your doctor's answers, instructions, and other appointment notes.

SET UP FILES

You will receive a lot of paperwork: lab results, healthcare bills, insurance statements, pamphlets, and more. On page 8 you will find a list of files to set up early on. This will help you be organized so that you will not be swamped with paperwork or stressed later on looking for information.

Long after treatments end, *The Breast Cancer Companion* will be a valuable record of your medical care and a roadmap for your follow-up care and recovery. The **Recovery** chapter provides an outline for you to discuss plans with your healthcare team for your follow-up care, your nutrition, an exercise plan, and stress-reduction techniques. In the **My Team and My Plans** chapter, you will find a 6-year planner that is perfect for keeping you on track with recommended checkups and screenings.

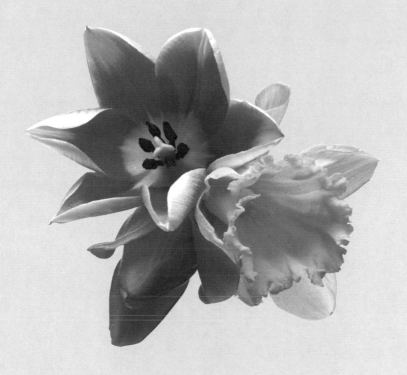

First Steps

First Steps

When learning of a diagnosis of breast cancer, it is very natural to feel overwhelmed. At first, there is so much information to digest along with a rollercoaster of emotions that it can be difficult to focus clearly.

Many women who have been diagnosed with breast cancer and their doctors share the following important advice: Take a deep breath!

In the beginning, you have *time* to learn about your diagnosis and explore treatment plans. It is very easy to want to rush to do something, but you have time to get the facts and consider your choices. Gather all the needed information from your medical team, Internet searches, books, organizations, and friends.

This may mean getting a second opinion and maybe even a third opinion. Your goal is to confirm the diagnosis and believe that the treatment plan that *you* choose is your best option.

Before the First Consultation

Soon, you will meet with your doctor to discuss your diagnosis. Much of the information about your diagnosis will come from a combination of **imaging techniques**, a **biopsy** of the breast tissue, and a laboratory analysis that will be summarized in a **pathology** report, which is described in detail later in this chapter.

What are imaging techniques? Imaging techniques, such as mammograms, ultrasound, MRI, and CT scans are used to help determine the size and extent of the cancer.

> *"Understand that it is normal to be afraid. Allow yourself to process the fear, to cry, to rage—whatever you need so that you can move to action. Action—making appointments, scheduling surgery, etc. gives you control."*
>
> **Claudia Francoeur**
> 3-YEAR SURVIVOR

Examples of Imaging Techniques

Mammogram—X-ray of the breast.

Breast Ultrasound—Additional view of a small area of the breast. It can show whether a lump is solid or filled with liquid.

Breast Magnetic Resonance Imaging (MRI)—Provides a high-resolution look at the breast without radiation.

Computed Tomography (CT) Scan—Can detect extremely small tumors that may not be seen on an x-ray.

Position Emission Tomography (PET) Scan—Used to determine if cancer cells have spread outside of the breast. Radioactive sugar is placed in a vein. A special camera makes detailed pictures of the places where the sugar collects.

Bone Scan—Used to check if the breast cancer has spread to the bones.

Chest X-ray—Used to see if the breast cancer has spread to the ribs or lungs.

What is a biopsy? A biopsy is performed to remove a tissue sample from the area of question in the breast. The tissue sample is sent to the lab and examined to determine whether it is cancerous. Breast biopsy is done by a specially trained radiologist or surgeon. There are four biopsy techniques: needle, stereotactic needle, incisional, and excisional.

A pathologist will prepare a **pathology report** to describe the specific disease characteristics of the cancer and will tell you and your doctor what kind of cancer you have. The type of breast cancer you have determines your individual treatment options.

> *"The surgeon I chose planned a visit and sat down with me and my husband. Her first words were 'we have a lot to discuss and I'm here to answer all your questions.' I knew I had the right physician from the moment I called for an appointment. The staff was kind, courteous and responsive right from the beginning."*
>
> **Elizabeth Lewis**
> 10-YEAR SURVIVOR

Step 1   Initial Consultation With Your Doctor

○ Review the **pathology report** carefully with your doctor. The pathology report is described in detail later in this chapter.

○ Ask your doctors for a copy of all tests and lab results. This will be helpful as you seek out additional opinions and meet new doctors. In addition, you will have a lifetime record of your care.

○ Your doctor will direct you to a breast surgeon (or surgical oncologist) for surgical treatment to remove the cancer. There are usually at least two surgical options. To select a surgical oncologist, network for names. Ask your primary care doctor, gynecologist, friends, family, and other medical professionals for recommendations of surgeon(s) with whom you can discuss your surgical options.

Step 2   Get Organized

In the coming weeks, you will be asked to fill out many forms and you will be asked for the same information repeatedly. Make this less stressful for yourself by filling out the following forms in this book. Bring this book to every appointment. Make copies of the forms in this book to hand out at your appointments.

- ○ **Medical History.** Fill out your medical history and your family's medical history (both father's and mother's families), especially because it relates to cancer. A medical history form is found on page **110**.
- ○ **Medications.** List the prescriptions, over-the-counter drugs, and supplements that you are currently taking. Fill out the **Medication Log** on page **113**.
- ○ **Insurance Information.** Fill out your health insurance information on page **123**.
- ○ **Emergency Contacts.** Fill in your emergency contact information on the inside front cover of this book.

Step 3   Build Your Team

- ○ **Pick a Buddy.** Many women have found it extremely valuable to have a friend, family member, spouse, or partner accompany them to every doctor visit. Your **buddy** can take notes, listen when you have stopped listening, and help you digest the doctor's recommendations. In these early meetings, doctors have a lot of information to share and it is really important to have someone with you who will be actively taking notes. If your buddy cannot make it to a doctor visit, consider bringing a tape recorder to the visit, in addition to note taking in the **Journal and Appointment Notes** section of this book.

- ○ Upon completion of your surgical treatment, your surgeon will refer you to a breast cancer oncologist. Individual circumstances may dictate that you see an oncologist before surgical treatment. Other medical professionals on your team may include:

    Medical Oncologist—Diagnoses and treats cancer with medicines, such as chemotherapy, hormonal therapy, and biologic therapy.

    A Breast Health Navigator—A certified nurse who collaborates with your doctor, your treatment team, and other resources, allowing you to focus on one thing—your health.

    Oncology Nurse—Administers chemotherapy. An oncology nurse is specially trained to help you deal with the emotional and physical side effects of breast cancer treatment.

    Radiation Oncologist—Specializes in treating cancer through radiation techniques.

    Reconstructive Surgeon—Specializes in breast reconstruction after mastectomy.

    Educationally Focused Support Groups—Provides information and guidance about breast cancer, treatment options, and the recovery process.

    The **My Team Directory** in this book is a convenient place for you to keep track of names, phone numbers, business cards, and appointment slips.

_____
_____
_____
_____
_____
_____
_____
_____
_____
_____
_____
_____
_____
_____
_____
_____
_____
_____
_____
_____
_____
_____

"In choosing a medical team, it was very important for me to have physicians who were willing to talk with me and answer all my questions. I had referrals from my internist, gynecologist, and friends. It was the longest two days of life when I was trying to get appointments and to find a doctor."

Elizabeth Lewis
10-YEAR SURVIVOR

Step 4 Insurance

○ Call your insurance company about requirements for referrals; some companies require that you see a gynecologist or an internist before seeing a cancer specialist. Without this referral, you may have trouble getting reimbursement for needed testing and treatments.

○ Ask about coverage for second opinions. Ask if your insurance company will provide you with a case manager to help you understand your benefits and coordinate your plan coverage. For a helpful guide and a list of questions to ask your insurance company, see page **124**. Having this information now will put your mind at ease and avoid issues later about procedures and reimbursements.

○ List your insurance information on page **123**. You will be asked for this information again and again.

○ If you do not have insurance, ask if your hospital has a social worker who can speak to you about financial issues. For a list of resources for financial aid for treatments and prescription medicine, see page **122**.

Step 5 Get Information

In the next few weeks, you will decide on a treatment plan. It is very important that you feel confident that this plan will be successful. It is essential that you feel you have explored available options.

○ As noted earlier, get a copy of your pathology report. Have a medical professional review your pathology report with you. See page **9**, **Understanding the Pathology Report**, for a glossary of the terms you will find in the report.

○ You may want to get a *second opinion*. Your goal for the second opinion is to confirm that you have breast cancer, confirm the type and nature of the cancer, and explore what other treatment plans are recommended for you to consider.

  ● Use the **Second Opinion Guide** on page **21** to help navigate the second opinion process.

○ If need be, get a third opinion. When recommendations differ considerably, you may feel you need a third opinion to help you decide on the course of treatment that is best for you.

○ Research the latest information that is available from your doctor and from the Internet. In the **Resources** chapter of this book, you will find a listing of helpful organizations, books, magazines, and Web sites.

○ Get a copy of *Breast Cancer Clear and Simple* from the American Cancer Society (*www.cancer.org*). This complete and easy-to-understand book subtitled *All Your Questions Answered* will be a welcomed resource in the first weeks after your diagnosis.

Step 6 Set Up Files

You will quickly be inundated with lots of paper: test results, bills, statements, receipts, claims, and explanations of benefits from every doctor, specialist, hospital, and treatment center that is part of your health care. In addition, you will be given or will pick up brochures, pamphlets, and news articles.

Our advice is that you set up a filing system early on. Set aside a filing drawer or buy a portable accordion file or large three-ring binders from an office supply store.

Setting up these files will save you time in the future and will help you feel organized and in control.

> *"Don't feel pressured or rushed into making treatment decisions. Do your research, interview more than one doctor for each specialty."*
>
> **Lynn Duchan**
> 3-YEAR SURVIVOR

Here are the file labels that will be useful for your file folders:

○ **Diagnostic Tests**—Use this folder to store a copy of your pathology, imaging, operative reports, as well as Onco*type* DX, Adjuvant! Online, and other report summaries.

○ **Medical and Lab Tests**—Request copies of all test results as the information develops. DO NOT WAIT. Test results are owned by you. Copies generated as they occur are not a burden for the medical staff to produce. Having this information for reference in the future will be valuable.

○ **Instructions From My Doctor**—Store notes from your doctor, such as preoperative instructions, your nutritional plan, recommended resources, etc., in this folder.

○ **Insurance**—Store medical insurance statements, medical insurance correspondence, and claim reimbursement explanations here in this folder.

○ **Bills and Medical Expenses**—Store your receipts for medical expenses, medical bills, and out-of-pocket travel expenses. For tax purposes, keep a record of vehicle mileage.

○ **Hospital Forms and Pamphlets**—Store news clippings, articles, pamphlets, and hospital brochures that you want to save.

○ **Prescriptions**—Drop your package inserts or drug description handouts from the pharmacy in this folder for later reference. You can use this information to help complete the **Medication Log** in this book. You will be asked to tell each of your doctors about all the prescriptions, over-the-counter drugs, and supplements you are taking, as well as any allergies you have. Bring this folder to your pharmacist or doctor if you have questions about your medications. It is recommended that you read the potential side effects so that you know what to expect and when to call your doctor.

○ **Research and Clinical Trials**—There is new information every month about treatments for breast cancer. Share this information with your doctor. Your doctors may have special insight about these new items and recommendations.

> *"When I am called by a woman who is newly diagnosed with breast cancer, my first words are 'Don't be afraid.'"*
>
> **Shelly Kassen**
> 7-YEAR SURVIVOR

Long after treatments end, *The Breast Cancer Companion* will be a valuable record of your medical care and a roadmap for your follow-up care and recovery.

Understanding the Pathology Report

The pathology report provides key information from the laboratory examination of the tissue sample from a breast biopsy or surgery. By law, you are entitled to a copy of your pathology report. This report describes what type of cancer you have and the extent of the cancer. Your doctors will use this information to design your individual treatment plan.

It is important that you review the pathology report with your doctors and maintain a copy of it for your records. Store your pathology report in your folder entitled Diagnostic Tests.

Questions You May Have for Your Doctor About Your Pathology Report

What kind of breast cancer do I have?

What is the stage of this type of breast cancer?

What is the grade and what does that mean?

May I have my breast biopsy reviewed by a pathologist at another diagnostic center?

What other studies are done on my tissue?

Do these study results define my treatment?

The pathology report will generally contain the following sections:

- **Personal Information**—Name, date of birth, date of the biopsy, and other identifying information.
- **Clinical History**—Information about what symptoms led to the biopsy and the type of surgery that was done to obtain the sample tissue.
- **Clinical Diagnosis**—The doctor's diagnosis before the breast tissue sample was tested.
- **Gross Description**—The size, weight, and color of the sample and any other features that the pathologist observed with the naked eye.
- **Microscopic Description**—Features of the cells as observed under a microscope, including:
  - Size of the tumor.
  - **Invasiveness**—Is the cancer intact (noninvasive), in a duct or lobule (in situ), or has the cancer broken the wall of a duct or lobule and become invasive?
  - **Grade**—Several different rating scales are used to describe numerically how closely the cancer cells resemble normal cells. The grade is a measure of the rate of growth of the cancer cells. Your doctor can explain the scale used by the pathologist.

- **Margin**—The pathologist will look at the margin around the tumor to determine whether it is clear of cancer cells. If the margin shows cancer cells, another surgery may be necessary to remove more tissue to get to a clear margin.

- **Lymph Node Status**—Reports whether the cancer has spread into the lymph nodes. Doctors also look at the amount of cancer in the lymph nodes. Here are the terms used to identify lymph node status:
  - ☐ **Microscopic**—Only a few cancer cells are in the node. A microscope is needed to find them.
  - ☐ **Gross**—There is a lot of cancer in the node. You can see or feel the cancer without a microscope.
  - ☐ **Extracapsular Extension**—Cancer has spread outside the wall of the node.

- **Lymphovascular Invasion**—Reports whether the cancer has spread into the blood vessels or lymph channels. There are two types of lymph nodes, sentinel and axillary. If cancer is found in the sentinel node biopsy, then axillary nodes will also be biopsied.

- **Special Tests or Markers**—Reports the results of tests for hormones, proteins, genes, and how the cells are growing and how fast. This information, specifically about human epidermal growth factor receptor 2 (HER2) status, estrogen receptor (ER) status, and progesterone receptor (PR) status will guide treatment options.

- **Summary and Diagnosis**—This part of the report summarizes the findings of the tests and categorizes the type of breast cancer that was found.

  The more common **types of breast cancer** are:

  ### Noninvasive Types

  Ductal Carcinoma In Situ (DCIS) refers to breast cancer that is in the breast's milk ducts, the tiny tubes that bring milk from where it is manufactured (in the lobules) to your nipple. It is the most common type of noninvasive breast cancer.

  Lobular Carcinoma In Situ (LCIS) is NOT cancer, but it is a sign that the woman who has it is six to seven more times likely to develop cancer over the course of her lifetime than a woman who does not have LCIS—the same risk you would have if your mother and sister both had cancer.

  ### Invasive Types

  Infiltrating Ductal Carcinoma (IDC) is the most common type of breast cancer; 70% of women with breast cancer have this diagnosis.

  Invasive/Infiltrating Lobular Carcinoma (ILC) occurs in the milk-producing lobules. Although most breast cancer (86% of all breast cancer) occurs in the ducts, just 12% occurs in the lobules. Lack of a palpable lump is one aspect of lobular cancer distinguishing it from ductal (*www.healthcentral.com*).

Inflammatory Breast Cancer (IBC) is a rare aggressive form of breast cancer not usually detected by mammograms or ultrasounds. This type of breast cancer is called *inflammatory* because the breast often looks swollen and red, or inflamed. IBC requires immediate aggressive treatment with chemotherapy prior to surgery and is treated differently than more common types of breast cancer.

Less common types of invasive breast cancer are medullary carcinoma, tubular carcinoma, colloid or mucinous carcinoma, and papillary carcinoma.

Following the biopsy and other necessary treatment or surgery, a pathology report will indicate the stage of the cancer. The **stage** of the cancer is a shorthand way to describe how big the tumor is and how far it has spread, and is a key factor in what treatment is recommended.

Here are the pathological stages of breast cancer as described in the brochure *Surgery Choices for Women with Early-Stage Breast Cancer* (US Department of Health and Human Services, National Institute of Health and the National Cancer Institute.[*www.cancer.gov/cancertopics/breast-cancer-surgery-choices*]).

Stage 0:

This means that you have either DCIS or LCIS. DCIS is very early breast cancer that is often too small to form a lump. LCIS is not cancer, but may increase the chance that you will get breast cancer. Talk with your doctor about treatment options if you are diagnosed with LCIS.

Stage I:

Your cancer is less than 1 inch across (2 cm) or about the size of a quarter. The cancer is in the breast and has not spread to lymph nodes or other parts of your body.

Stage IIA:

☐ No cancer is found in your breast, but cancer is found in the lymph nodes under your arm;

☐ Your cancer is 1 inch (2 cm) or smaller and has spread to the lymph nodes under your arm; or

☐ Your cancer is about 1 to 2 inches (2–5 cm) but has not spread to the lymph nodes under your arm.

Stage IIB:

☐ Your cancer is about 1 to 2 inches (2–5 cm) and has spread to the lymph nodes under your arm; or

☐ Your cancer is larger than 2 inches (5 cm) and has not spread to the lymph nodes under your arm.

Stage IIIA:

- ☐ No cancer is found in the breast but is found in lymph nodes under your arm, and the lymph nodes are attached to each other;

- ☐ Your cancer is 2 inches (5 cm) or smaller and has spread to lymph nodes under your arm, and the lymph nodes are attached to each other; or

- ☐ Your cancer is larger than 2 inches (5 cm) and has spread to lymph nodes under your arm.

Stage IIIB:

This means there is a tumor of any size that has grown into the chest wall or the skin of the breast. It may be associated with swelling of the breast or with nodules (lumps) in the breast skin.

- ☐ The cancer may have spread to lymph nodes under the arm.

- ☐ The cancer may have spread to underarm lymph nodes that are attached to each other or other structures, or the cancer may have spread to lymph nodes behind the breastbone.

- ☐ The cancer is inflammatory breast cancer (IBC), a rare type of breast cancer. The breast looks red and swollen because cancer cells block the lymph vessels in the skin of the breast. When a doctor diagnoses IBC, it is at least Stage IIIB, but it could be more advanced.

Stage IIIC:

This means there is a tumor of any size and it has spread in one of the following ways:

- ☐ The cancer has spread to the lymph nodes behind the breastbone and under the arm.

- ☐ The cancer has spread to the lymph nodes above or below the collarbone.

Late-stage breast cancer, or invasive breast cancer is described as:

Stage IV:

Invasive cancer—The breast cancer has spread beyond the breast to other parts of the body (such as bone, lung, liver, or brain).

Deciding on a Treatment Plan

Every patient and every breast cancer is unique. The best and optimal treatment plan often is a combination of different therapies. There may be more than one treatment approach that will be appropriate. In general, there are two types of therapy for breast cancer: **local** and **systemic**.

Local Therapies

Local therapies are used, first, to remove the cancer from the breast, surrounding tissue, and lymph nodes and second, to treat the site of the cancer. Examples of local treatments are **surgery** and **radiation**.

Surgery. The goal of surgery is to physically remove the cancer from the breast.

Radiation. This therapy uses high-energy x-rays, which are applied to very small areas of the breast or lymph nodes to prevent the cancer cells from growing. There are two types of breast radiation. External radiation is most commonly administered after a lumpectomy. Internal radiation, the delivery of radioactive seeds via catheters, is currently in research studies.

> *"Learn as much as possible about your breast cancer so that you can make informed decisions and have a sense of control in these stressful times."*
>
> **Elizabeth Lewis**
> 9-YEAR SURVIVOR

Surgery Choices. The National Cancer Institute has produced a very helpful brochure, *Surgery Choices for Women with Early-Stage Breast Cancer* that is a very good resource for comparing the different breast cancer surgery options. This brochure may be found at your medical center and/or can be viewed online at *www.cancer.gov*.

Types of Breast Cancer Surgery

Breast-Sparing Surgery—Means that the surgeon removes only the cancer and some normal tissue around it. This type of surgery keeps your breast intact—looking a lot like it did before surgery. Lumpectomy, partial mastectomy, breast conserving surgery, or segmental mastectomy are all considered breast-sparing surgery.

Lymph Node Biopsy—A sentinel lymph node biopsy is done to ascertain whether the cancer has spread beyond the breast tissue. Sentinel lymph node removal has a minimal risk of a potentially painful side effect called lymphedema. An axillary lymph node dissection is a surgical procedure that removes additional lymph nodes if the cancer is found to have spread in any of the sentinel lymph nodes.

Mastectomy Surgery—Means that the surgeon removes all of your breast and nipple. Here are some types of mastectomy.

- ○ **Total (simple) mastectomy.** The surgeon removes your entire breast. Sometimes, the surgeon also takes out some of the lymph nodes under your arm.
- ○ **Modified radical mastectomy.** The surgeon removes your entire breast, many of the lymph nodes under your arm, the lining over your chest muscles if the tumor is attached to the muscle, and maybe a small chest muscle.

○ **Double mastectomy.** The surgeon removes both breasts at the same time, even if your cancer is in only one breast. This surgery is rare and mostly used if there is a high risk that you might develop cancer in the other breast.[1] You may choose this for nonmedical reasons, such as:

- Genetic presence of either the breast cancer 1 (BRCA1) or breast cancer 2 (BRCA2) gene.
- Concern/fear for a second cancer in a healthy breast.

Not all mastectomies are medically necessary. You have the right to choose a mastectomy to further reduce your risk of recurrence. Your decision of whether to get a mastectomy (with or without reconstruction) will be influenced by your body perception, age, marital status, and concern for risk of another breast cancer. The decision to have a double mastectomy should not be done as a reflex action. Make sure that you clarify all of your options.

Reconstructive Surgery (surgery to rebuild the breast)—Your treatment plan may call for surgery to remove a breast or to remove a breast lump. Removal of a lump from a small breast may alter the breast contour, in which case you may decide to have some reconstruction performed. The unaffected breast can be considered for reconstruction as well.

With removal of a breast, you can choose simultaneous (a one-step procedure) or delayed reconstruction. You will want to have a discussion with your doctors about what is right for you. Your doctors will guide you through your options based on your health, treatment plan, and goals.

○ Discuss options and timing with your doctors. Reconstruction options are:
- Breast implant
- Latissimus dorsi flap
- Transverse rectus abdominus muscle flap
- Mammoplasty

○ Interview plastic surgeons.

○ Health insurance companies that cover mastectomies must also cover costs for reconstruction and prostheses. This coverage is guaranteed by law through the Women's Health and Cancer Rights Act. Contact your insurance company to understand what will be covered. Find out if there is a difference in coverage based on the types of reconstruction, and whether the reconstruction is done right away or is delayed.

○ For a comprehensive explanation of the breast reconstruction process, read *The Well-Informed Patient's Guide to Breast Reconstruction*, by Stephen Kroll, M.D. The book is online and provides a detailed look at the results of surgery using diagrams that outline the reconstructive process, as well as before and after photographs taken of actual patients (*www.mdanderson.org/diseases/breastcancer/reconstruction*).

---

[1] Adapted from the brochure *Surgery Choices for Women with Early-Stage Breast Cancer*, US Department of Health and Human Services, National Institute of Health and the National Cancer Institute (2004).

○   *The Breast Reconstruction Guidebook* (second edition) by Kathy Steligo is another resource that is highly recommended by breast cancer patients. This book explains the benefits and limitations of each reconstructive technique, and what to expect at each step of the way: before your surgery, in the hospital, during recovery, and life beyond reconstruction.

Questions to Ask your Doctor About Reconstructive Surgery

What types of breast reconstruction are available? What are the advantages and disadvantages of each choice?

What does each type of reconstruction involve? How long is the process? Are there multiple surgeries? Are the surgeries done on an inpatient or outpatient basis?

How many of each procedure have you performed? With all of the procedures available, what is your specialty?

Why are you recommending a particular reconstruction for me over the other options? (Note: A surgeon may only recommend the procedure he or she is most familiar with. It is important for you to learn about all reconstruction options, including no reconstruction, so that you can make the best informed decision for yourself.)

What is the latest information about breast implants? What are you recommending? Why?

With reconstruction, can I change the size of the breasts? Can both breasts have reconstruction?

How will the reconstructed breast feel to the touch? Will there be any feeling (sensation)?

Can I see photographs of other patients who have had breast reconstruction? Do you have any former/current patients I can speak to? (Note: Federal privacy laws prohibit your doctor from giving out a patient's name and phone number without permission. Some doctors have thoughtfully obtained such permission and can have a former or current patient contact you so you may learn about the surgery and recovery from the patient's perspective.)

Are there specific techniques that could benefit me if further treatments are needed, such as radiation?

Systemic Therapies

Systemic therapies are used to get rid of cancer cells that may be in the bloodstream, lymphatic system, or by direct extension into surrounding tissue, and may have travelled to other sites in the body, such as the bones, liver, lung, or brain. Examples of systemic therapies are:

Chemotherapy. This therapy uses combinations of drugs to kill cancer cells throughout your body.

Hormonal Therapy. Some breast cancers, those that are ER-positive or PR-positive grow faster when certain hormones are present. Hormone therapy reduces the production of these hormones to prevent the tumor cells from growing.

Tumors can be tested at the time of surgery for hormone receptors to see if they can be treated with hormones. The most commonly used hormone therapy is the drug **tamoxifin**. Another group of drugs used for estrogen positive postmenopausal women is **aromatase inhibitors**. Your oncologist will evaluate your tumor pathology for this treatment.

Targeted Biologic Therapies. Biologic therapy can work by boosting the patient's immune system. Biologic therapies such as trastuzumab (Herceptin) attach to the cancer cells to stop or slow their growth.

Clinical Trials

A clinical trial is a medical research study in which participants volunteer to test new methods to prevent, screen, diagnose, or treat a disease. The goal of these projects is to find safe, more effective treatments for patients. Should a new treatment prove effective, patients in this trial are the first to receive the resulting treatment.

There are four phases of cancer clinical trials.

Phase	Trial Purpose
I	Evaluate Safety
II	Measures Effectiveness
III	Tests Against the Best Existing Treatment
IV	Evaluates New Uses or Long-Term Effects of the Treatment

How to Find a Clinical Trial

Fortunately, there are fabulous resources today to help you and your doctor find out about clinical trials that may be relevant and available for your situation.

- The Coalition of Cancer Cooperative Groups is a superb source for up-to-date cancer clinical trial information through TrialCheck, a free online matching system. TrialCheck, winner of the 2008 Consumer Health World Award "Best in Show," links patients, caregivers, and the health care community to unbiased cancer clinical trials by matching relevant cancer trials to patients by filtering information such as type of cancer, zip code, and other criteria (*www.cancertrialshelp.org* or call 1-877-520-4457).

- The National Cancer Institute (NCI) has tens of thousands of clinical trials in progress at any one time. You can find information about cancer trials run by NCI online at *www.cancer.gov/clinicaltrials* or by calling the NCI Information Service at 1-800-4-CANCER (1-800-422-6237).

- The American Society of Clinical Oncology (ASCO) is the voice of the world's cancer physicians. ASCO has created an oncologist-approved Web site for patients, *www.cancer.net*. This valuable Web site for patients that provides in-depth information about clinical trials, resources for finding an oncologist, patient stories, and guides to help you make the decision of whether to participate in a clinical trial (*www.cancer.net*/patient or call 1-571 483-1300).

CLINICAL TRIALS TO DISCUSS WITH MY DOCTOR

Name of study _____

Phase of trial _____

Research organization _____

Eligibility requirements _____

_____

Contact (phone/Web) _____

_____

Name of study _____

Phase of trial _____

Research organization _____

Eligibility requirements _____

_____

Contact (phone/Web) _____

Name of study _____

Phase of trial _____

Research organization _____

Eligibility requirements _____

_____

Contact (phone/Web) _____

Clinical Trial Terminology

Bias—When a point of view prevents impartial judgment on issues relating to the subject of that point of view. In clinical studies, bias is controlled by blinding and randomization.

Blind—A randomized trial is blind if the participant is not told which arm of the trial he or she is on. A clinical trial is blind if participants are unaware on whether they are in the experimental or control arm of the study.

Control Group—The standard by which experimental observations are evaluated. In many clinical trials, one group of patients will be given an experimental drug, whereas the control group is given either a standard treatment for the illness or a placebo.

Double-Blind Study—A clinical trial design in which neither the participating individuals nor the study staff knows which participants are receiving the experimental drug and which are receiving a placebo (for another therapy).

Informed-Consent Document—A document that describes the rights of the study participants, and includes details about the study, such as its purpose, duration, required procedures, and key contacts. Risks and potential benefits are explained in the informed-consent document. The participant then decides whether to sign the document. Informed consent is not a contract, and the participant may withdraw from the trial at any time.

Placebo—A placebo is an inactive pill, liquid, or powder that has no treatment value. In clinical trials, experimental treatments are often compared with placebos to assess the treatments' effectiveness.

Randomization—A method based on chance by which study participants are assigned to a treatment group. Randomization minimizes the differences among groups by equally distributing people with particular characteristics among all the trial arms. The researchers do not know which treatment is better. From what is known at the time, any one of the treatments chosen could be of benefit to the participant.

Excerpted from *www.clinicaltrials.gov/ct2/info/glossary*.

Genetic Testing: Is It Right for Me?

During your consultations with your doctor, you will review your family history of cancer. Your doctor may advise that you be referred to a certified genetic counselor to consider being tested for the presence of the BRCA1 or BRCA2 gene. Researchers have determined that approximately 5% to 10% of women with breast cancer have a hereditary form of the disease and that the inherited alterations in the genes called BRCA1 and BRCA2 are involved in many cases of hereditary breast cancer.

> "The likelihood that breast cancer is associated with BRCA1 or BRCA2 is highest in families with a history of multiple cases of breast cancer, cases of both breast and ovarian cancer, one or more family members with two primary cancers (original tumors at different sites), or an Ashkenazi (Eastern European) Jewish background. However, **not every** woman in such families carries an alteration in BRCA1 or BRCA2, and not every cancer in such families is linked to alterations in these genes." (NCI, *www.cancer.gov*)

The presence of BRCA1 or BRCA2 may influence treatment recommendations and the choices about your treatment. If you have concerns about possible repercussions as a result of genetic testing, you should be aware of Genetic Information Nondiscrimination Act (GINA), a federal regulation that prohibits health insurance discrimination based on genetic testing and/or information. In addition, many states have laws protecting against genetic discrimination as well. Your certified genetic counselor can give you more information about this important topic.

If you need more information or assistance finding a certified genetic counselor, visit NSGC.org, the Web site for the National Society of Genetic Counselors (NSGC).

For support and information, visit FORCE (Facing Our Risk of Cancer Empowered), an organization dedicated to providing resources for women at risk of hereditary breast cancer resulting from family history or BRCA genetic status at *www.facingourrisk.org*.

For More Help With Making Your Treatment Decision

The **National Comprehensive Cancer Network** (NCCN) is an alliance of 21 of the world's leading cancer centers, working together to develop treatment guidelines for most cancers, and dedicated to research that improves the quality, effectiveness, and efficiency of cancer care. NCCN offers a number of programs to help you and your family make informed decisions about your health.

NCCN offers patient-friendly summaries to educate patients about the latest available treatments for their disease and prepare patients to talk to their doctors about the therapies that may be right for them (*www. nccn.com*).

In addition, there are two services that can help you and your medical team decide on an optimal treatment plan. They are **Adjuvant! Online** and **Onco*type* DX**.

Ask your doctors for access to the following services. Because of the complexity of interpretation of some of the input information (ambiguities about tumor size, margins, etc.), the information *should be entered* by a health professional who has experience in cancer medicine.

- **Adjuvant! Online.** Have your medical oncologist register for Adjuvant! Online. The purpose of Adjuvant! Online is to help health professionals and patients with early cancer discuss the risks and benefits of getting adjuvant therapy, such as chemotherapy, hormone therapy, or both after surgery (*www.adjuvantonline. com*).

- **Onco*type* DX.** It is a genomic test that examines tumor genes and estimates the risk of future recurrence. Onco*type* DX is a clinically validated laboratory test, ordered by authorized health care providers, that predicts the likelihood of breast cancer recurrence in women with newly diagnosed, early stage invasive breast cancer.

  Currently Onco*type* DX also assesses the benefit of chemotherapy for women with ER-positive and node-negative pathology (*www.genomichealth.com*).

Second Opinion Guide

You may want to get a second opinion. To start, you may want a second doctor to confirm the initial diagnosis. Look for a doctor who is at a medical center that has a lot of experience in breast cancer and an expert pathology reputation.

Start this process as soon as possible. Your first doctor will understand that you want additional input and can help you make the calls to arrange for the second opinion consultation.

"No Travel" or "Remote" Second Opinions

There is a way to get a second opinion from some of the top medical centers in the country without leaving home. Through a relatively new type of consultation called *online second opinion services*, you arrange to have your medical records sent to one of these services. Within 1 to 2 weeks, you will receive recommendations from one of the country's top specialists regarding your treatment.

The advantages to these services are that you can eliminate the time and expense of travel to these medical centers **and** you have access to expert advice quickly. These services cost between $500 and $1500 and are generally not covered by insurance. There are three main leaders in "remote" second opinion services: Partners Online Specialty Consultations, eCleveland Clinic, and Johns Hopkins Medicine International. In each of these cases, these services are from hospitals that rank at the top of *U.S. News & World Report* magazine's *The Best of the Best* for cancer care.

○ **Partners Online Specialty Consultations.** The consultation process is managed by Center for Connected Health and draws on the expertise of the physicians of all of the Partners hospitals including Brigham and Women's Hospital, Massachusetts General Hospital, and Dana-Farber/Partners CancerCare (*https://econsults.partners.org*).

○ **eCleveland Clinic** is a Web-based extension of the Cleveland Clinic. MyConsult, eCleveland Clinic's service, provides patients with online second opinions, health news, and health information regardless of their location.

The Cleveland Clinic will ask for actual films or studies that are deemed necessary for eCleveland Clinic physicians to perform a thorough assessment. Patients print a customized checklist from the Web site and request these items from the doctor or hospital where the patient's tests were performed

You can register on the eCleveland Clinic Web site at *www.eclevelandclinic.org*.

○ **Johns Hopkins Medicine International's** remote medical second opinion program allows you to consult with a Johns Hopkins specialist to confirm your diagnosis, review your current treatment plan, and discuss possible treatments at Johns Hopkins. As with the other remote second opinion services, you and your physician will have the advantage of a valuable resource for staying up to date on the latest research and therapeutic advances for your condition (*www.jhintl.net*).

First Opinion Record

Doctor _____

Referred by _____

Phone number_____ Fax _____

Address _____

Report and records sent _____ Received _____

PROCEDURE FOR SENDING RECORDS

Send reports

_____ Breast imaging reports (i.e., mammogram, ultrasound, and MRI)

_____ Pathology report

_____ Operative report if surgery has been performed

_____ Recent lab results

_____ Any previous treatment records, if applicable

Send pathology slides. (Pathology slides are irreplaceable, so you may choose to hand deliver or send via a priority mail service.)

_____ Biopsy

_____ Lumpectomy

_____ Mastectomy

Send imaging films

_____ Mammogram, ultrasound, MRI

_____ Other imaging films such as PET, CT, bone scan, nonbreast MRI, and chest x-ray as requested.

Will an independent pathologist review pathology slides? _____

Will an independent breast radiologist review imaging records? _____

Does the doctor agree with the diagnosis? _____

Date of consultation _____

Recommendation for treatment _____

_____

_____

_____

_____

Second Opinion Record

Doctor _____

Referred by _____

Phone number_____ Fax _____

Address _____

Report and records sent _____ Received _____

PROCEDURE FOR SENDING RECORDS

Send reports

_____ Breast imaging reports (i.e., mammogram, ultrasound, and MRI)

_____ Pathology report

_____ Operative report if surgery has been performed

_____ Recent lab results

_____ Any previous treatment records, if applicable

Send pathology slides. (Pathology slides are irreplaceable, so you may choose to hand deliver or send via a priority mail service.)

_____ Biopsy

_____ Lumpectomy

_____ Mastectomy

Send imaging films

_____ Mammogram, ultrasound, MRI

_____ Other imaging films such as PET, CT, bone scan, nonbreast MRI, and chest x-ray as requested.

Will an independent pathologist review pathology slides? _____

Will an independent breast radiologist review imaging records? _____

Does the doctor agree with the diagnosis? _____

Date of consultation _____

Recommendation for treatment _____

_____

_____

_____

_____

Second Opinion Record

Doctor _____

Referred by _____

Phone number_____ Fax _____

Address _____

Report and records sent _____ Received _____

PROCEDURE FOR SENDING RECORDS

Send reports

_____ Breast imaging reports (i.e., mammogram, ultrasound, and MRI)

_____ Pathology report

_____ Operative report if surgery has been performed

_____ Recent lab results

_____ Any previous treatment records, if applicable

Send pathology slides. (Pathology slides are irreplaceable, so you may choose to hand deliver or send via a priority mail service.)

_____ Biopsy

_____ Lumpectomy

_____ Mastectomy

Send imaging films

_____ Mammogram, ultrasound, MRI

_____ Other imaging films such as PET, CT, bone scan, nonbreast MRI, and chest x-ray as requested.

Will an independent pathologist review pathology slides? _____

Will an independent breast radiologist review imaging records? _____

Does the doctor agree with the diagnosis? _____

Date of consultation _____

Recommendation for treatment _____

_____

_____

_____

_____

My Treatment Plan

Date

SURGERY PLAN

_____
_____
_____
_____
_____
_____
_____
_____
_____
_____
_____

CHEMOTHERAPY PLAN

_____
_____
_____
_____
_____
_____
_____
_____
_____
_____
_____
_____
_____

continues

My Treatment Plan

Date

RADIATION PLAN

OTHER THERAPY

6

THE BREAST CANCER COMPANION

My Treatment Plan

Date

RECONSTRUCTION

NUTRITION

REHABILITATION

Prepare for Surgery

Your doctor and nurse will give you very specific instructions on what to do, what not to do, and what to bring to your surgery. Create a folder entitled **Instructions From the Doctor** as a convenient place to keep these instructions. Here are some other things to consider that might make your hospital stay more comfortable.

- Pack a bag for hospital stay if you will be staying overnight in the hospital.
  - Robe (with big, roomy sleeves)
  - Slippers or no-slip socks (many hospitals provide cozy no-slip socks)
  - Makeup
  - Hair brush, comb
  - Toothbrush, toothpaste, floss
  - Relaxation materials (books, magazines, music, etc.)
  - Lip balm
  - Phone numbers
  - Reading glasses. If you wear contact lenses, you may not be permitted to wear them during surgery. Check with your doctor, and, if necessary, bring your glasses.
  - Cell phone and cell phone charger
  - Pen and notebook
  - Insurance card(s) and photo ID. Many hospitals require a photo ID at admissions.
  - A written list of current medications
  - A small travel pillow (10" × 10") to cushion surgical area
  - This book!
- Wear comfortable pants and a loose, front-opening top for returning home.
- Review postsurgery instructions with your doctor and your home caregiver.
- Ask your doctor if there is a formal pretreatment presentation for you to attend at your medical center.

Resource tip: Ask your surgeon or surgery nurse about obtaining a Necessities Bag before mastectomy surgery. The Necessities Bag is a reusable tote containing practical information, bandages, and essentials for wound care, hygiene, and personal comfort. This invaluable tote is distributed for free by a medical professional. It was created by Maureen Lutz whose surgical experience gave her perspective on how she should have prepared for her personal needs in the hospital and afterward at home (*www.necessitiesbag.org*).

Prepare Your Home for Recovery After Surgery

○ Fill *prescriptions* and have them ready at home. If you do NOT have small children at home, consider asking the pharmacist to eliminate the childproof caps, because you may have reduced strength when you first come home.

○ Set up your *nightstand* with things that you will need during the first few days that you are back at home:

- Telephone
- Reading material
- TV remote
- Soft tissues, hand lotion
- Phone numbers of doctors, family, and friends
- Water bottle or water pitcher

○ Use a postsurgical bra that is soft, front-fastening, with no underwire. Check with your doctor if you need to bring this bra to the hospital.

○ Be sure to wear button-front pajamas because you may find putting clothing on over your head uncomfortable.

○ If you are having a transverse rectus abdominis myocutaneous (TRAM) flap or latissimus dorsi flap reconstruction, you may find a recliner comfortable for postsurgical sleeping.

○ Line up your *caregivers*. This is the time to let others support you so that you can focus on your recovery. Discuss with your doctor what needs and limitations you will have during these first couple of weeks after surgery. Depending on the extent of your surgery, helpers could be necessary.

If a friend has offered to coordinate meals and errands, there are some fabulous Web sites available to organize your "help team." These free Web sites are ideal for scheduling and sharing information and messages (*www.lotsahelpinghands.com*, *www.carecalendar.org*, *www. whatfriendsdo.com*).

○ Prepare and freeze your favorite foods ahead of time. Stock your home with normal foods.

○ Set up friends and family to help with your children's transportation, activities, and home routine for your first few days home.

○ Sign up a friend as your "mass communicator." Make up an e-mail list of family and friends who will want to know about your treatments and progress.

○ CaringBridge is a free Web site that helps keep loved ones informed through a patient journal. Family and friends give patient and caregiver support through guestbook messages (*www.caringbridge.org*).

> *"Take care of yourself first. . . This is the time to focus on you. . . . Allow others to help, whether it's bringing a meal, picking up groceries, or driving you somewhere. It's a gift to your friends to let them help you. It gives others a chance to help you in your fight."*
>
> **Claudia Francoeur**
> 4-YEAR SURVIVOR

Prepare for Chemotherapy

When and How

Chemotherapy is a treatment with drugs. In the case of breast cancer, these are drugs that kill cancer cells and are given as pills, capsules, or liquid form, injected in a vein (intravenously), and through a new method called heat therapy.

Chemotherapy is usually given in a clinical setting, a hospital, doctor's office, or cancer treatment center. It is administered for several cycles. The total length of your treatment will depend on the chemotherapy drugs in your plan.

If your treatment is given intravenously, your doctor may recommend that you have a **port** inserted in your chest wall to make the chemotherapy easier and more comfortable for you. A port is inserted in a simple, same-day surgery and removed after all the cycles of chemotherapy treatment are finished. Using a port eliminates the need to use a vein and can be used for blood tests.

Tip: Ask your doctor for a prescription for a numbing ointment for the site of the port. This is usually applied to the skin directly over the port 1 hour before treatment, eliminating discomfort.

Questions You May Have for Your Doctor About Chemotherapy treatments:

When will treatment start? End? How often will I have treatment?

How will chemotherapy affect my daily life?

How will I know that the treatment is working?

Are there any special services for patients?

What antinausea drugs are available and how do I get them?

Plan Ahead

Before you start chemotherapy, your doctor will explain what side effects you might expect from the treatments. Each drug has different side effects and each person reacts differently. Some typical side effects experienced are hair loss, fatigue, nausea, mouth sores, fever, and sickness. On a positive note, there are new drugs and treatment plans to lessen the intensity of these side effects. Once you know what to expect, it helps to be prepared. Here are some things that you can do ahead of time:

O Arrange for someone to help organize volunteer help for family activities— carpooling, meals, grocery shopping, and babysitting around the time of treatment.

O Fill any prescriptions in advance for treating side effects.

O Do NOT take any alternative medicines or supplements without discussing with your oncologists.

O Have a good thermometer on hand.

○ Schedule a complete dental exam and cleaning prior to chemotherapy. This is a preventive procedure to avoid unnecessary risk of infection.

○ If it is near the time for your annual Pap smear (cervical cancer screening test), consider having a Pap smear done before treatments begin. Chemotherapy can cause abnormal results.

○ If your doctor has indicated that you will lose your hair, you may consider:

- Shopping for a wig before hair loss. It is ideal because you can match up your hair color and style beforehand. If your budget permits, you may consider buying a second wig as backup while the first is being washed or styled (see **Resources** chapter).

- Shop for hats and/or head scarves for protection from the weather. Tip: Beanie hats are great for sleep time.

- Cutting your hair before it falls out. Many professional wig makers will be able to style a natural-looking wig with your own hair. You can also have a ponytail or bangs made from your own hair or to wear under a hat or scarf. See Hip Hats With Hair (*www.hiphat.com*), for cute ways to have hair without wearing a wig.

- Many insurance companies will pay for a wig (it may be referred to as a cranial prosthesis). Check with your insurance company if you will need a prescription first. Several organizations provide wigs at no charge, including the American Cancer Society, Cancer Cares, and the Breast Cancer Network of Strength. For more information, refer to the **Resources** chapter in the back of this book.

- Consider attending a local **Look Good . . . Feel Good** workshop, which teaches beauty techniques to help restore one's appearance and self-image during chemotherapy and radiation treatments. Lessons are offered one-on-one or in hands-on workshops, and include a 12-step skin care/make up application lesson, demonstration of options for dealing with hair loss, and nail care techniques. You will receive personal advice from certified cosmetologists and take home complimentary cosmetic kits and advice about wigs, scarves, and accessories (*www.lookgoodfeelbetter.org*).

When to Call the Doctor?

Discuss with your doctor reasons to call such as side effects including those that you did not expect, shaking chills or fever, unusual cough, sore throat, lung congestion or shortness of breath, vomiting, or inability to eat or drink for more than 24 hours. In addition, your doctor wants you to call when:

_____

_____

_____

_____

_____

During Treatments

Treatments, particularly those that are given on a slow-drip intravenous method, can take anywhere from one to several hours.

To pass the time during your chemotherapy treatments, you may want to bring the following:

- A friend
- A good book or magazines
- Your laptop computer
- Music with headphones
- Notepaper for writing letters
- Relaxation techniques, such as guided imagery or visualization and progressive muscle relaxation and meditation, have proved to be effective in lessening anxiety and side effects. Find a technique and practice it to use during your chemotherapy sessions.
- Snacks!

"Take it one day at a time. Focus on yourself and getting better."

Linda Ruberto
11-YEAR SURVIVOR

Managing Side Effects From Chemotherapy

Your doctor and oncology nurse may have some recommendations for relief from side effects. Here are some tips that have helped other women deal with and sometimes prevent side effects:

"Plan something special for yourself for after a treatment . . . lunch with a friend, a walk, yoga, a funny movie."

Karen Como
6-YEAR SURVIVOR

- A **metallic aftertaste** is common after some chemotherapy drugs. Eat foods such as pretzels, tart hard candies, dry crackers, lemonade, tea, and starchy foods.
- **Mouth sores.**
  - Try rinsing with saltwater or baking soda mixtures.
  - Use a prescription numbing agent, like Xylocaine.
- **Dry mouth.** Biotene Gel or Biotene Dry Mouth Toothpaste, Oral Balance, and Biotene Gum help to increase saliva flow. Find these in your local pharmacy or at *www.dentist.com* or *www.drugstore.com*.

○ **Nausea.** Your doctor should outline a plan prior to chemotherapy so that you are prepared if nausea occurs. Ask your doctor about antinausea medications. Drinking lots of fluid, before and after a chemotherapy session, seems to help with nausea. Try eating plain foods such as crackers and dry toast, sipping on clear beverages, and eating popsicles and Jell-O. Some patients have found relief from nausea with a combination of acupuncture and medications.

○ **Dry skin.** Moisturize after your shower or bath. Use moisturizing body wash instead of soap. Use hand lotion frequently.

○ **"Chemo brain."** Some women experience "chemo brain," where you find that you are unable to concentrate on your work, lose your train of thought, stumble on words, or are unable to juggle multiple tasks. You may find that you do not remember things as well as you used to. Speak to your doctor about these symptoms. He or she may want to rule out other causes. In the case of chemo brain, treatments may include medication, stimulants, exercise, and more reliance on planners and other aids.

○ **Hot flashes.** Chemotherapy-induced menopause can be temporary or permanent depending on the patient's age at the start of treatment. Hot flashes are a common symptom of menopause. Hot flashes occur when estrogen is blocked in the hypothalamus, the part of the brain that controls the thermostat. There are a variety of ways to treat hot flashes. Your medical team can help you find an effective and acceptable remedy.

> *"Set goals for yourself to get through the next week. Know that you will get back your regularly scheduled life."*
>
> **Shelly Kassen**
> 7-YEAR SURVIVOR

The ABCs of Blood Cell Counts

Chemotherapy and radiation can cause a **decrease** in your normal blood cells. A complete blood count (CBC) measures your blood cell levels. Your blood cells have important functions:

- White blood cells (WBCs) fight infection.
- Platelets (PLTs) help stop bleeding by clotting the blood.
- Red blood cells (RBCs) carry oxygen to all parts of your body.
- Hemoglobin in the RBC carries the oxygen.

Tip: Request copies of your blood work lab tests for your files. Keep a record of your blood tests in the Medical and Lab Results record on page **117**. It is important for you to track your results.

> "My blood counts never recovered after chemo. Same has been true with others I have spoken with. You will want to have a history of this all in one place."
>
> **Eileen Margherio**
> 4-YEAR SURVIVOR

During your chemotherapy treatments, protect yourself from infection by avoiding people with infection, colds, and contagious diseases, and by washing your hands repeatedly during the day.

Call your doctor right away if you have any of the following signs of an infection or any symptoms that seem unusual or concerning to you:

- Temperature over 100°F
- Shaking chills
- New dry or moist cough
- A burning feeling when urinating
- Loose bowels
- Sore throat
- Flu-like symptoms
- Any skin rash

Lab tests explained. Here are two good resources for helping you understand the numbers behind your lab tests.

www.Labtestsonline.org is a brilliant Web site designed to help you better understand the many clinical lab tests that are part of routine care as well as diagnosis and treatment of a broad range of conditions and diseases. One can search by condition, such as breast cancer, or by a specific test.

In addition, The Leukemia & Lymphoma Society has produced a booklet, *Understanding Lab and Imaging Tests*. To order your free copy, call 800-955-4572 or go to *www.lls.org*.

Prepare for Radiation Treatments

○ **Schedule** the radiation planning appointment. You may choose to bring someone with you to this meeting for listening purposes. Treatment decisions will be made at this consultation.

Questions You May Have for Your Doctor About Radiation Treatments

What is radiation therapy?

What risks or side effects are there with radiation?

When will the radiation treatments occur and for how many weeks?

What is used for marking the radiation treatment area?

What should I do to get ready for the treatments?

How will radiation treatments affect my daily life?

Will radiation be painful? Will it cause any scarring?

Are there any special services for patients undergoing radiation treatment?

○ During treatment, **wear clothing** that is loose and easy to get off and on. Choose tops that are soft (like pima cotton) and lightweight, as your skin is likely to be tender during the course of treatments. Choose cotton bras or T-shirts and camisoles that will not further irritate sensitive skin.

○ **Very important!** Skin care needs to start after the very **first** radiation treatment to prevent skin reactions.

○ Avoid **skin products** such as soap, deodorant, talcum powder, perfumes, and lotions before treatment sessions. Some ingredients in these products may further irritate sensitive skin in the treatment area and interfere with the radiation beams. Discuss these precautions with your radiation therapist.

○ Reactions from radiation range from the sensation of mild sunburn to redness, peeling, and blistering. Be prepared to get products to soothe your skin and help with the healing process. Speak to your radiation nurse about recommended products for you, such as:

> **Salves** such as aloe vera, Calendula ointment, Aquaphor, Lubriderm, or Biafine
>
> **Gel pads** or gel sheets such as Radiacare gel sheets for cooling the burn.
>
> **Burn ointments** and a nonstick covering, such as Telfa pads, when the skin is blistering.

○ Have **sunscreen** (SPF 30 +) on hand to protect your skin, as the radiation sites will be very sensitive to sun exposure for the next year. **Note:** No sun exposure is allowed for 1 year on the breast area that was radiated.

○ Develop some positive healing thoughts for your radiation treatments. Use positive visualization techniques, such as imagining that the radiation beams are zapping the cancer cells.

○ As the radiation treatments go on, you may experience some **fatigue**. This may be a good time to call on your family and friends for support.

○ Schedule an appointment with a nutritionist. Certain foods can help you feel less tired during radiation treatments, especially high-protein foods. For examples, see page **48** in the **Recovery** chapter of this book.

○ Attend an educationally focused breast cancer support group for information, networking, and support.

"A support group was instrumental to help me understand and cope with everything emotionally."

Gail Johnson
6-YEAR SURVIVOR

Reconstruction and Prosthesis

If you choose reconstructive surgery:

○ Your doctors will give you specific instructions on how to prepare for surgery. Mark your planning calendar for any appointments and medical tests before and after the reconstruction surgery.

○ Your instructions may include filling prescriptions and buying supplies, as well as guidelines on eating and drinking, smoking, and taking or avoiding certain vitamins and medications.

○ Ask your doctor if it will be necessary to arrange for someone to help you for a few days after the surgery.

○ If you are a smoker, you must stop smoking before your surgery. Discuss this with your surgeon.

○ Review the **Prepare Your Home for Recovery After Surgery** checklist.

If you choose breast prosthesis:

After your treatments, you may choose not to have additional surgery for reconstruction. In this case, an alternative option is to use a breast prosthesis. A breast prosthesis (or breast form) is most often made of silicon and is designed to be worn inside your bra to resemble the weight and natural contour of your breast.

There is an extensive range of breast prostheses available today. If carefully fitted, no one would know that you are wearing breast prostheses under your clothes.

Medical specialty stores, lingerie stores, hospital shops, and some larger department stores offer a broad range of bra styles and prostheses. Be sure there is a fitter available to help you with your selection. Mail order supplies are not recommended as an individual fitting is a must. Your oncologist or surgeon can give you a prescription (for insurance purposes) and recommendations for where to shop nearby.

Here are some tips for getting a breast prosthesis:

○ Find out what is covered by your health insurance company.

○ Find a source near you that has trained fitters who can help you with your selection. Call for an appointment.

○ Wear a T-shirt or form-fitting shirt so that you can see that the fit looks natural. Walk around the store for 30 minutes or more to make sure that you are comfortable with the fit.

○ You can adapt your bras with pockets to hold the prosthesis or buy special bras (and swimsuits!) that have built-in pockets.

○ Medicare/Medicaid and most major health insurance companies provide postsurgical bras and prostheses at no charge. Contact your insurance carrier for your personal coverage.

○ Several organizations may provide prostheses at no charge, including the American Cancer Society, Cancer Cares, and the Breast Cancer Network of Strength organization. For more information, refer to the **Resources** chapter of this book.

I Have Kids!

If you have children, you are probably wondering what to tell them, how to say it, and just how much information your children need. Each woman needs to follow her own heart and do what is right for her family.

Most experts advise that what children generally need most is **honesty**, **reassurance**, and, as best as you are able, **a normal routine**. There are wonderful resources online that provide guidance to parents with cancer, especially for parents of teens. Here are a few tips about talking with children about cancer.

It is best for you to be the one tell the children about the cancer. Plan the conversation in advance and choose a time when the whole family can be together. It is best to tell them as soon as you are ready because children at all ages will pick up quickly that something is wrong. Often they will imagine the worst.

> **Younger children**—Use simple language that is in their vocabulary. Most agree that it is important to name the sickness as "cancer." Prepare the children for expected side effects and explain that this is from the strong medicine that is helping *get rid of the cancer*.
>
> Younger children may have separation fears, so it is helpful to have familiar caregivers stay with them should you have to stay in the hospital.
>
> Reassure children that their needs will be met.
>
> Let your children know that cancer is not contagious.
>
> Encourage your children to ask you questions. This way you will be better able to understand any fears or concerns that they have.
>
> **Teenagers**—In addition to your honesty and reassurance, older children are more likely to know more about cancer from school and from the media. If they do not ask, they may be wondering about survival rates and specifics about your treatment and side effects.
>
> **Teenage Girls**—Be aware that your teenage daughter may have special concerns. In a recent survey, BreastCancer.org found that nearly 30% of teenage girls feared that they had breast cancer. Although the risk of young women developing breast cancer is very small, there is a lot of publicity about celebrities with breast cancer and breast cancer awareness in general. You may want to address this concern directly.
>
> Marissa Weiss, MD, the founder of BreastCancer.org wrote *Taking Care of Your Girls: A Breast Health Guide for Girls, Teens, and In-Betweens* (Three Rivers Press, 2008) to help educate young women about breast health. This chatty and informative guide for moms and their teenage girls is accompanied by a Web site for girls: *www.takingcareofyourgirls.com*.

Again, as well as possible, maintain your usual family routine. Be sensitive that your teenagers may wonder whether it is okay for them to proceed with normal activities. It is likely that they will be called on to help more at home, and they may need permission to continue with their schoolwork, sports and other activities, and time with their friends.

Your family will all benefit from trying to maintain as normal a family routine as you are able. This is a great time to let friends and family help with meals, rides and other chores, and babysitting.

Let the other adults in your children's lives know what is going on, including caregivers, teachers, school counselors, coaches, and parents of your children's friends as you feel is appropriate.

Resources

There are several books and Web sites that offer advice and excellent tips for coping with family matters while you are being treated for breast cancer. Here are a few:

Books

Talking to Kids About Cancer. Cancer Patient Care (Dana Farber Cancer Institute, 2008).

When a Parent Has Cancer: A Guide to Caring for Your Children. Wendy S. Harpham (Harper Paperbacks, 2004). Written by a mother, physician, and cancer survivor, this highly praised book provides practical advice on caring for children of all ages during diagnosis and treatment.

Web site

www.breastcancer.org/tips/telling_family/, which is part of the **Breastcancer.org** Web site under Day-to-Day matters. Breastcancer.org provides an in-depth guide on how to help your children understand and cope when a parent has cancer.

Organization

CancerCare provides telephone education workshops connecting cancer experts from around the country to families affected by cancer. CancerCare also offers the following booklet: *Helping Children When a Family Member Has Cancer*. A printable version is available online at *www.cancercare.org*.

In addition, you may be able to find a support group for your children in your area by contacting your local chapter of the American Cancer Society or speaking with hospital social workers, nurses, psychologists, clergy members, and school counselors.

I Have a Husband/Partner!

If you are married or in a committed relationship, your husband/partner is likely to be deeply affected by your diagnosis with breast cancer. Understandably, at this time, much of the focus and attention is on you, your needs, and your emotions. If your roles were reversed, you can imagine how worried and helpless you would feel. Dealing with cancer is very stressful and can be stressful on your relationship with your husband/partner.

Here are a few things to consider:

○ Guide your husband/partner as to how much or how little to help! Husbands/partners may go into fix-it mode or, on the other extreme, retreat from the situation. Discuss with your husband/partner about what is the right balance of intervention. Be clear about your needs and when you want to handle issues yourself.

○ Talk to your husband/partner about his or her feelings. It is important to share and support each other. Recognize that your coping styles may be very different. Your husband/partner may be anxious about any number of issues: being a good caregiver, fear of losing you, disrupted routines, financial issues, or other concerns.

○ Include your partner in medical appointments and treatments when possible. Your husband/partner will hear the information first-hand and be in a better position to help you with decisions and dealing with side effects.

Get help if you are having trouble talking with your partner about your cancer. Find support from others—your doctor, social worker, therapist, or couples support group. In addition, your husband/partner may find the following resources helpful:

Men Against Breast Cancer (MABC) is a national nonprofit organization designed to provide support services to educate and empower men to be effective caregivers. MABC created a book called *For the Women We Love: A Breast Cancer Action Plan and Caregiver's Guide for Men*. To order this book and for other support resources, go to *www.menagainstbreastcancer.org*.

Breast Cancer Network of Strength provides a unique service for those who are supporting a woman through breast cancer—the **Partner Match Program**. The program provides support and education for people while they are supporting a wife, partner, or other loved one through the disease. The **Partner Match Program** matches you with a person who has had similar experiences being the caregiver or loved one of a survivor. Simply call the YourShoes 24/7 Breast Cancer Support Center at 1-800-221-2141 (*www.networkofstrength.org*).

Books

Breast Cancer Husband: How to Help Your Wife (and Yourself) During Diagnosis, Treatment and Beyond by Marc Silver (St. Martin's Press, 2004).

Diary of a Breast Cancer Husband by J. Scott Lyman (Times Publishing Group, 2002).

Helping Your Mate Face Breast Cancer by Judy C. Kneece (EduCare Publishing, 2001).

I Have a Job!

One of your many concerns after a diagnosis of breast cancer is how to handle your job. Talk with your doctor about your job and how the treatments will affect you. Some women feel best keeping a normal life as before the diagnosis, and are able physically and emotionally to continue at their work. Other women may choose to focus completely on their family and their recovery. The only answer here is what feels best for you and your situation.

Some of the questions you may have are:

Should I tell my boss and coworkers about my breast cancer diagnosis?

> You will probably want to tell your boss if you will be taking time off from work for appointments and treatments. Otherwise, your commitment and productivity may be questioned. You may choose to tell your coworkers who share responsibilities with you, so that they understand your absences. If you are comfortable, you may choose to tell everyone at work.

What if I am treated differently at work because of my health condition?

> There are laws to protect you from discrimination because of a health issue, but only if your employer is aware of your condition. If you feel that you have been treated unfairly, contact the US Equal Employment Opportunity Commission (EEOC) through their Web site at *www.eeoc.gov* for more information about your rights.

Could I lose my job if I have to take time off?

> Talk to your boss about how much time you expect to need. Keep a record of your talks with your boss and with the benefits people at your job. In the event that you are threatened with dismissal, you may have protection under the Americans with Disabilities Act (*www.ada.gov*). If your company is larger than 50 employees, you are guaranteed up to 3 months of unpaid time to take care of yourself through the Family and Medical Leave Act (FMLA) (*www.dol.gov/esa/whd/*).

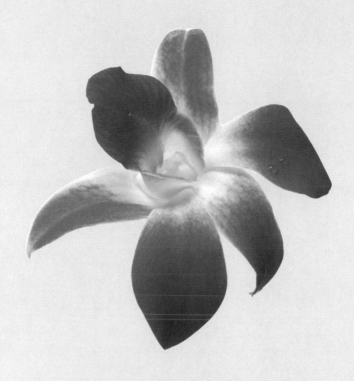

Recovery

FEEL BETTER BY LIVING WELL

Follow Up With Your Doctors

Eat Well

Vitamins, Minerals, and Herbs

Be Physically Active

Reduce Stress

Sexuality and Intimacy

Feel Better by Living Well

Once your treatments have ended, you will no longer have the regimen of treatment appointments and doctor visits to guide your care. The best thing you can do is to shift your focus to living a healthy lifestyle and being diligent in your follow-up care as recommended by your doctor. Taking steps to live well is a good way for all women to help increase their chance of remaining cancer free.

Studies have shown that diet and exercise contribute to breast cancer survival. Significantly, a recent study shows that breast cancer survivors who eat a healthy diet and exercise moderately can reduce their risk of dying from breast cancer by half, regardless of their weight.[1]

Here is what you can do to live well and stay well:

- Follow up with your doctors as recommended by your medical team.
- Eat well.
- Be physically active.
- Reduce stress.
- Enjoy sex and intimacy.
- Do not smoke.
- Manage your weight.
- Move on with life's interests. You are a survivor.

"Every day is a blessing. Live life to the fullest. Stay in the moment!!!"

Linda Ruberto
11-YEAR SURVIVOR

"It will get better. There will be a time when your cancer no longer consumes your life."

Lynn Duchan
3-YEAR SURVIVOR

"It takes a while to feel "normal." Don't try to rush it."

Claudia Franceour
4-YEAR SURVIVOR

---

[1] This study was done by the Moores Cancer Center at the University of California, San Diego (UCSD) and published in the June 10, 2007 issue of Journal of Clinical Oncology.

"Exercise daily!"

Eileen Margherio
4-YEAR SURVIVOR

"Don't try to overdo during and after treatment/surgery. Allow yourself time to grieve, to recover, to renew. Reach out to friends and family and doctors for support as needed."

Lynn Duchan
3-YEAR SURVIVOR

"I attended support groups during and after treatment. I highly recommend it. It was a tremendous support for me. There were people who shared the same diagnosis, and I didn't have to filter any thoughts or feelings. Most important, I didn't feel alone and knew there were others to help me on my road to recovery. As they say, priceless."

Elizabeth Lewis
10-YEAR SURVIVOR

"Become involved with breast cancer fundraising. This is a good way to give back for all the support that you received."

Shelly Kassen
7-YEAR SURVIVOR

"Don't be afraid to say 'no.' Allow your body, mind and sprite the time it needs to recover. There comes a day when breast cancer isn't in your thoughts."

Claudia Franceour
4-YEAR SURVIVOR

"Find your passion. . . and do it!"

Catherine Stone
8-YEAR SURVIVOR

Follow Up With Your Doctors

After your treatments end, make an appointment with your oncologist and primary physician to discuss your follow-up schedule. Use the **Planning Calendar** in this book to map out your appointments. Save time by booking your appointments all at one time so that you have peace of mind knowing that you have everything scheduled.

Although you are probably weary of doctor appointments and medical tests, it is important that you also remain vigilant with your regular health screening tests. Speak to your primary physician for a recommendation on how often to have the following screening tests.

O Digital mammogram—This can be self-referred. Have this ONLY at an accredited radiological center.

O Pap smear test

O Cholesterol check

O Blood pressure

O Colorectal cancer test

O Diabetes

O Depression

O Osteoporosis

O Immunizations

O Skin cancer screening

O Dental exams

> *"Be vigilant and don't miss appointments. Keep yourself up on all the latest breast cancer findings."*
>
> **Eileen Phelps**
> 16-YEAR SURVIVOR

Speak to your oncologist about what symptoms to be alert for and when to contact your doctor. Your doctor may have you call if you notice changes in your breasts, bone pain, skin rashes, chest pain, weight loss, or other changes. Record these below.

If you had an axillary node dissection, talk with your doctor about **lymphedema**. Swelling of your arm and extremities can be potentially painful and may occur years after your surgery. **Note:** Your doctor may prescribe compression sleeves and/or special exercises to prevent and treat lymphedema. For more information, refer to the National Lymphedema Network, *www.lymphnet.org* or call the hotline at 1-800-541-3259.

Tip: Space your follow-up appointments with your surgeon, medical oncologists, and primary doctor so that you are being evaluated on a regular basis during the year. The 6-year Planning Calendar in this book is a convenient place to plan these screenings.

SYMPTOMS: Your doctor wants you to call if you notice the following symptoms or changes:

_____
_____
_____
_____
_____
_____
_____

Eat Well

Nutrition plays a key role in your ongoing health, managing side effects, and in the strength of your immune system. Speak with your doctor for nutrition recommendations. Your doctor may refer you to a registered dietitian for a specific plan tailored to your health goals and needs.

In general, your goal is to eat a healthy diet and maintain a normal weight.

Healthy Eating Guidelines

○ Follow a balanced diet with a **variety** from the main food groups.

○ With your doctor's approval, increase your daily protein. Protein-rich foods include beef, pork, chicken, fish, eggs, lentils, and yogurt. Protein is an important nutrient for rebuilding healthy cells.

○ Eat five to seven servings of daily **fruits and vegetables**.

○ Emphasize foods that are **whole grain** when choosing cereals, breads, rice, pasta, and other grain products.

○ Choose **low-fat** dairy products.

○ Choose **leaner meats**, limiting processed and red meat.

○ Drink lots of **water**.

○ Drink little or no alcohol.

○ Soy products of any kind are **NOT** recommended.

NUTRITION RECOMMENDATIONS FROM YOUR HEALTH TEAM:

Vitamins, Minerals, and Herbs

During treatment for breast cancer, dietary supplements of vitamins, minerals, and herbs should only be taken upon the advice and/or with the consent from your doctor. Your doctor will consider underlying health conditions (such as diabetes or high blood pressure), the treatment drugs that you are (or will be) taking, and supporting research before recommending a supplement to your nutrition plan.

Some dietary supplements can work against breast cancer treatment and can interfere with the way prescription medicine works. Therefore, it is vital that you consult with your doctor before taking any supplements during your treatment and recovery.

Make sure you disclose any supplements you are taking to your doctor!

Women undergoing treatment for breast cancer can experience significant bone loss because of anticancer drugs. In these cases, your doctor and registered dietitian will recommend food sources for calcium and vitamin D, and may recommend dietary supplements to support bone health.

DIETARY SUPPLEMENT RECOMMENDATIONS FROM YOUR
HEALTH TEAM:

_____
_____
_____
_____
_____
_____
_____
_____
_____
_____
_____
_____
_____
_____
_____
_____
_____
_____
_____
_____
_____
_____
_____
_____
_____
_____
_____
_____
_____
_____
_____
_____
_____
_____

Be Physically Active

You can make a difference in your well-being by increasing your physical activity. Moderate, daily exercise is good for you in all kinds of ways: it improves your mood, increases your energy, relieves stress, strengthens your muscles and bones, helps to lower blood pressure, improves cholesterol levels, and more! Studies show that exercise is important for breast health and lowering breast cancer risk as well.

Before you begin, talk to your doctor about starting an exercise program.

Make exercise part of your daily routine. Exercise can be any physical activity that gets you moving such as walking, dancing, working in the yard, or working out at the gym.

Schedule your exercise just like any other appointment, whether it is a walk in the neighborhood or a session with a personal trainer.

Change it up! Try different activities until you find that perfect combination of things that you enjoy, that keep you interested, and that keep you moving! Doing different activities throughout the week has the added benefit of working different muscles and building up your flexibility, endurance, and strength.

As you are putting together your plan, you will want to incorporate cardiovascular workouts, stretching, strength training, and balance into every week. *The Breast Cancer Survivor's Fitness Plan*, by Carolyn M. Kaelin, MD, MPH (McGraw-Hill, 2007) is a wonderful guide to help you choose effective exercises based on the type of surgery that you have had and your fitness level. Dr. Kaelin is the director of the Comprehensive Breast Health Center at Brigham and Woman's Hospital, which is associated with Harvard Medical School, as well as a breast cancer survivor herself.

Ideas for adding more physical activity:

- Exercise with a friend.
- Keep a written log of your schedule and your accomplishments!
- Have a back-up plan for bad weather.
- Invest in a pedometer (which counts your footsteps).
- Include music in your workout.
- Plan active weekends (walks, hikes, biking).
- Be active throughout the day! If you need to, divide up your total daily exercise time and do them at different parts of the day.
- Walk instead of drive whenever possible.
- Take the stairs instead of the elevator or escalator.
- Park at the far end of the parking lot.
- Walk a few blocks before getting on the bus.
- Take a 10-minute walk after lunch.
- Walk your dog.
- Garden, rakes leaves, or do some house cleaning every day.
- Wash and wax your car by hand.

YOUR EXERCISE PLAN:

_____

_____

_____

_____

_____

_____

_____

_____

_____

_____

_____

_____

_____

_____

_____

_____

_____

_____

_____

_____

_____

_____

_____

_____

_____

_____

_____

_____

_____

_____

_____

_____

Reduce Stress

A wealth of research has demonstrated that stress weakens the immune system. You can benefit by taking steps to reduce stress in your life during and after treatment for cancer. Reducing stress is considered so helpful that many cancer centers and hospitals around the country are offering complementary therapies that include support groups, music, art, movement, visualization, and meditation along with traditional cancer treatments.

What Can You Do?

Talk to your doctor or nurse about using stress therapy or "mind/body techniques" that may help to strengthen your immune system and assist your body in fighting the effects of the cancer.

Find a therapy that works for you. Try to spend 10 to 20 minutes each day on some form of deep relaxation. Some of the techniques to explore are:

- Meditation
- Visualization
- Yoga or Tai Chi
- **Deep Breathing Exercises.** Sit or lie down and uncross your legs and arms. Take in a deep breath. Then push out as much air as you can. Breathe in and out again, this time relaxing your muscles on purpose while breathing out. Keep breathing and relaxing for 5 to 20 minutes at a time.
- **Exercise.** Moving and stretching your body is a great stress reliever. A daily walk might do the trick.
- **Progressive Relaxation Therapy.** Tense muscles and then relax them. Learn these techniques from a clinic or audiotape.
- **Remove Sources of Stress.** Identify and get rid of sources of stress in your life as best you can. If you cannot remove the stresses, try changing the way you think about them. Find ways to view the situation in a positive light.
- **Seek Support.** When you feel burdened by stress, find someone with whom you can share your concerns. (This may include a counselor or therapist.) Do not wait to feel overwhelmed. Locate a support group facilitated by a nurse that focuses on education after treatment is completed. To find a support group, contact your nearby hospital or the local chapter of the American Cancer Society.

Sexuality and Intimacy

Understandably, intimacy often goes to the bottom of the list when a woman is going through breast cancer treatments. Fatigue, body image, vaginal dryness, and your emotional psyche are factors that can discourage feeling and being sexual. Because sexuality and intimacy are personal expressions of one's self and one's relationship with others, sharing and closeness can be healthy and restorative at this time.

Body image issues loom large for many women. It is very normal to feel differently about your body when dealing with a diagnosis of cancer. This may be because of the loss of a breast in the case of a mastectomy, disruption or ceasation of your menstrual cycle, loss of sexual sensation, or because you just do not feel sexy at this time. As you are experiencing these changes, your partner may also be having anxieties as well. Both of you are adjusting. Therefore, it is important that you talk candidly about your feelings. Open communication between partners is part of an ongoing recovery to sexual health.

Where do you go for advice and encouragement? Because sexuality and intimacy issues are very common for women with breast cancer, there are a number of people on your medical team who can talk with you and give you suggestions for your situation. Start with the person on your team with whom you would be most comfortable opening up about your concerns. Consider discussing your situation with your gynecologist, a therapist or social worker, a sex therapist, or as part of your breast cancer support group.

Our sexuality is an important part of our lives and an important part of recovery.

Online resource: *www.breastcancer.org/tips/intimacy*

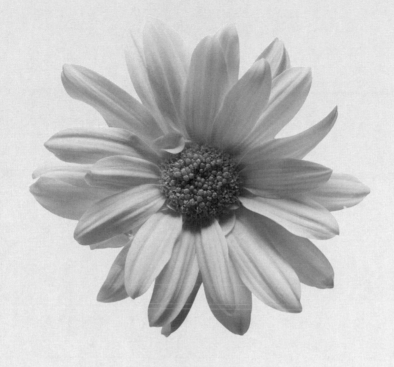

My Team and My Plans

TEAM DIRECTORY

PLANNING CALENDAR

JOURNAL AND APPOINTMENT NOTES

THANK YOU, THANK YOU! JOURNAL

My Team and My Plans

Team Directory

Here is a convenient place to keep track of the names and phone numbers of those very important people who make up your breast cancer support team.

Your breast cancer support team will include doctors, nurses, and other medical specialists, as well as family, friends, and support groups—all of whom will give you strength and support throughout your recovery journey. Use this directory to keep track of all your important numbers.

Your team may include:

Primary Physician—Provides you with regular medical care and will refer you to specialists.

Breast Health Navigator—A certified nurse who ensures that you receive the support and knowledge you need to successfully navigate the health care system.

The breast health navigator collaborates with your doctor, your treatment team, and other resources, allowing you to focus on one thing: your health.

Medical Oncologist—Diagnoses and treats cancer with medicines, such as chemotherapy, hormonal therapy, and biologic therapy.

Oncology Nurse—Administers chemotherapy. An oncology nurse is specially trained to help you deal with the emotional and physical side effects of breast cancer treatment.

Breast Surgeon/Oncologist Surgeon—Specializes in removing cancer through surgery.

Radiation Oncologist—Specializes in treating cancer through radiation techniques.

Plastic or Reconstructive Surgeon—Specializes in breast reconstruction after mastectomy.

Pathologist—Examines breast tissue in the laboratory in order to diagnose cancer and further analyzes the cells to determine the nature and extent of the cancer.

Physical Therapist—Trained to help you during your recovery.

Social Worker—Trained to talk with you and your family about the emotional challenges of breast cancer and to help you locate support services as needed.

Certified Genetic Counselor—Trained to assess and counsel you and your family about risks for hereditary cancer, including genetic testing for breast cancer genes.

> **Tip:** It can be a valuable time-saver for you to have the name and phone number of the staff in your doctor's office.
>
> **Your doctor's assistant (or administrator)** has access to your doctor's schedule and procedure scheduling.
>
> **Your doctor's medical assistant** can readily answer many of your medical questions and concerns.
>
> **Find out if your doctor's respond to e-mails from patients!** This may be a great way to get quick answers to your questions and concerns.

Team Directory

PRIMARY PHYSICIAN

Name _____ Phone _____

Organization/Office Name _____

Office Address _____

Primary Nurse _____ Phone _____

Assistant's Name _____ Phone _____

Fax _____ E-mail _____

BREAST HEALTH NAVIGATOR

Name _____ Phone _____

Organization/Office Name _____

Office Address _____

Primary Nurse _____ Phone _____

Assistant's Name _____ Phone _____

Fax _____ E-mail _____

MEDICAL ONCOLOGIST

Name _____ Phone _____

Organization/Office Name _____

Office Address _____

Primary Nurse _____ Phone _____

Assistant's Name _____ Phone _____

Fax _____ E-mail _____

ONCOLOGY NURSE

Name _____ Phone _____

Organization/Office Name _____

Office Address _____

Primary Nurse _____ Phone _____

Assistant's Name _____ Phone _____

Fax _____ E-mail _____

Team Directory

BREAST SURGEON/ONCOLOGIST SURGEON

Name _____ Phone _____

Organization/Office Name _____

Office Address _____

Primary Nurse _____ Phone _____

Assistant's Name _____ Phone _____

Fax _____ E-mail _____

RADIATION ONCOLOGIST

Name _____ Phone _____

Organization/Office Name _____

Office Address _____

Primary Nurse _____ Phone _____

Assistant's Name _____ Phone _____

Fax _____ E-mail _____

PATHOLOGIST

Name _____ Phone _____

Organization/Office Name _____

Office Address _____

Primary Nurse _____ Phone _____

Assistant's Name _____ Phone _____

Fax _____ E-mail _____

PLASTIC OR RECONSTRUCTIVE SURGEON

Name _____ Phone _____

Organization/Office Name _____

Office Address _____

Primary Nurse _____ Phone _____

Assistant's Name _____ Phone _____

Fax _____ E-mail _____

Team Directory

PHYSICAL THERAPIST

Name _____ Phone _____

Organization/Office Name _____

Office Address _____

Primary Nurse _____ Phone _____

Assistant's Name _____ Phone _____

Fax _____ E-mail _____

SOCIAL WORKER

Name _____ Phone _____

Organization/Office Name _____

Office Address _____

Primary Nurse _____ Phone _____

Assistant's Name _____ Phone _____

Fax _____ E-mail _____

CERTIFIED GENETIC COUNSELOR

Name _____ Phone _____

Organization/Office Name _____

Office Address _____

Primary Nurse _____ Phone _____

Assistant's Name _____ Phone _____

Fax _____ E-mail _____

Specialty _____

NUTRITIONIST

Name _____ Phone _____

Organization/Office Name _____

Office Address _____

Primary Nurse _____ Phone _____

Assistant's Name _____ Phone _____

Fax _____ E-mail _____

Specialty _____

Team Directory

Name _____ Phone _____

Organization/Office Name _____

Address _____

Fax _____ E-mail _____

Specialty _____

Name _____ Phone _____

Organization/Office Name _____

Address _____

Fax _____ E-mail _____

Specialty _____

Name _____ Phone _____

Organization/Office Name _____

Address _____

Fax _____ E-mail _____

Specialty _____

Name _____ Phone _____

Organization/Office Name _____

Address _____

Fax _____ E-mail _____

Specialty _____

Name _____ Phone _____

Organization/Office Name _____

Address _____

Fax _____ E-mail _____

Specialty _____

Name _____ Phone _____

Organization/Office Name _____

Address _____

Fax _____ E-mail _____

Specialty _____

Team Directory

Name _____ Phone _____

Organization/Office Name _____

Address _____

Fax _____ E-mail _____

Specialty _____

Name _____ Phone _____

Organization/Office Name _____

Address _____

Fax _____ E-mail _____

Specialty _____

Name _____ Phone _____

Organization/Office Name _____

Address _____

Fax _____ E-mail _____

Specialty _____

Name _____ Phone _____

Organization/Office Name _____

Address _____

Fax _____ E-mail _____

Specialty _____

Name _____ Phone _____

Organization/Office Name _____

Address _____

Fax _____ E-mail _____

Specialty _____

Name _____ Phone _____

Organization/Office Name _____

Address _____

Fax _____ E-mail _____

Specialty _____

Team Directory

Name _____ Phone _____

Organization/Office Name _____

Address _____

Fax _____ E-mail _____

Specialty _____

Name _____ Phone _____

Organization/Office Name _____

Address _____

Fax _____ E-mail _____

Specialty _____

Name _____ Phone _____

Organization/Office Name _____

Address _____

Fax _____ E-mail _____

Specialty _____

Name _____ Phone _____

Organization/Office Name _____

Address _____

Fax _____ E-mail _____

Specialty _____

Name _____ Phone _____

Organization/Office Name _____

Address _____

Fax _____ E-mail _____

Specialty _____

Name _____ Phone _____

Organization/Office Name _____

Address _____

Fax _____ E-mail _____

Specialty _____

Team Directory

Name _____ Phone _____

Organization/Office Name _____

Address _____

Fax _____ E-mail _____

Specialty _____

Name _____ Phone _____

Organization/Office Name _____

Address _____

Fax _____ E-mail _____

Specialty _____

Name _____ Phone _____

Organization/Office Name _____

Address _____

Fax _____ E-mail _____

Specialty _____

Name _____ Phone _____

Organization/Office Name _____

Address _____

Fax _____ E-mail _____

Specialty _____

Name _____ Phone _____

Organization/Office Name _____

Address _____

Fax _____ E-mail _____

Specialty _____

Name _____ Phone _____

Organization/Office Name _____

Address _____

Fax _____ E-mail _____

Specialty _____

Team Directory

Name _____ Phone _____

Organization/Office Name _____

Address _____

Fax _____ E-mail _____

Specialty _____

Name _____ Phone _____

Organization/Office Name _____

Address _____

Fax _____ E-mail _____

Specialty _____

Name _____ Phone _____

Organization/Office Name _____

Address _____

Fax _____ E-mail _____

Specialty _____

Name _____ Phone _____

Organization/Office Name _____

Address _____

Fax _____ E-mail _____

Specialty _____

Name _____ Phone _____

Organization/Office Name _____

Address _____

Fax _____ E-mail _____

Specialty _____

Name _____ Phone _____

Organization/Office Name _____

Address _____

Fax _____ E-mail _____

Specialty _____

Planning Calendar

Here is a convenient calendar for keeping track of your medical tests, scheduled treatments, and appointments.

After your surgery and radiation and/or chemotherapy treatments are completed, your doctors will recommend a schedule of follow-up tests and visits for probably several years. It is understandable that you may want to be free of doctors and appointments. However, it is very important that you are vigilant and follow-up with your oncologists and your other doctors. With this calendar, you can plan these important dates long in advance and review your appointments at a glance.

Tips:

○ Make notes on this calendar during your doctor visits.

○ From time to time, review this calendar with your doctors.

○ Schedule medical tests well enough in advance of doctor visits so that you can discuss the results in person.

○ Stagger your follow-up appointments with your surgeon, medical oncologist, and primary doctor, so that you are being frequently evaluated.

○ Use this calendar to coordinate for your regular health screenings as recommended by your oncologist and your other doctors:

- Mammograms—Only at a fully accredited radiological center
- Pap smear test
- Cholesterol check
- Blood pressure
- Colorectal cancer test
- Diabetes
- Depression
- Osteoporosis
- Immunizations
- Skin cancer screening
- Dental exams

Customizable Calendar

Month _____ Year _____

S	M	T	W	T	F	S

Month _____ Year _____

S	M	T	W	T	F	S

Month _____ Year _____

S	M	T	W	T	F	S

Month _____ Year _____

S	M	T	W	T	F	S

Month _____ Year _____

S	M	T	W	T	F	S

Customizable Calendar

Month _____ Year _____

S	M	T	W	T	F	S

_____
_____
_____
_____
_____
_____

Month _____ Year _____

S	M	T	W	T	F	S

_____
_____
_____
_____
_____
_____

Month _____ Year _____

S	M	T	W	T	F	S

_____
_____
_____
_____
_____
_____

Month _____ Year _____

S	M	T	W	T	F	S

_____
_____
_____
_____
_____
_____

Month _____ Year _____

S	M	T	W	T	F	S

_____
_____
_____
_____

Customizable Calendar

Month _____ Year _____

S	M	T	W	T	F	S

_____
_____
_____
_____
_____

Month _____ Year _____

S	M	T	W	T	F	S

_____
_____
_____
_____
_____

Month _____ Year _____

S	M	T	W	T	F	S

_____
_____
_____
_____
_____

Month _____ Year _____

S	M	T	W	T	F	S

_____
_____
_____
_____
_____

Month _____ Year _____

S	M	T	W	T	F	S

_____
_____
_____
_____

Customizable Calendar

Month _____ Year _____

S	M	T	W	T	F	S

_____
_____
_____
_____
_____

Month _____ Year _____

S	M	T	W	T	F	S

_____
_____
_____
_____
_____

Month _____ Year _____

S	M	T	W	T	F	S

_____
_____
_____
_____
_____

Month _____ Year _____

S	M	T	W	T	F	S

_____
_____
_____
_____
_____

Month _____ Year _____

S	M	T	W	T	F	S

_____
_____
_____
_____
_____

Customizable Calendar

Month _____ Year _____

S	M	T	W	T	F	S

_____
_____
_____
_____
_____
_____

Month _____ Year _____

S	M	T	W	T	F	S

_____
_____
_____
_____
_____
_____

Month _____ Year _____

S	M	T	W	T	F	S

_____
_____
_____
_____
_____
_____

Month _____ Year _____

S	M	T	W	T	F	S

_____
_____
_____
_____
_____
_____

Month _____ Year _____

S	M	T	W	T	F	S

_____
_____
_____
_____
_____
_____

Customizable Calendar

Month _____ Year _____

S	M	T	W	T	F	S

_____
_____
_____
_____
_____
_____

Month _____ Year _____

S	M	T	W	T	F	S

_____
_____
_____
_____
_____
_____

Month _____ Year _____

S	M	T	W	T	F	S

_____
_____
_____
_____
_____
_____

Month _____ Year _____

S	M	T	W	T	F	S

_____
_____
_____
_____
_____
_____

Month _____ Year _____

S	M	T	W	T	F	S

_____
_____
_____
_____
_____
_____

Journal and Appointment Notes

Use these pages for note taking during your appointments with your doctors. This is a good place to jot down questions for your doctor and to keep track of your own to do's such as scheduling follow-ups, prescriptions, and tests.

Plan to bring this journal to every appointment. You may also want to journal your treatment events and experiences by keeping appointment notes. Use the right hand column symbols so that you can easily skim your journal to find items for follow-up (☆), questions (?), and to check off items that are complete.

Date	Notes/Questions/To do's/Symptoms/Side effects	? Question ☆ To do

Date	Notes/Questions/To do's/Symptoms/Side effects	? Question ☆ To do

Date	Notes/Questions/To do's/Symptoms/Side effects	? Question ☆ To do

Date	Notes/Questions/To do's/Symptoms/Side effects	? Question ☆ To do

Date	Notes/Questions/To do's/Symptoms/Side effects	? Question ☆ To do

Date	Notes/Questions/To do's/Symptoms/Side effects	? Question ☆ To do

Date	Notes/Questions/To do's/Symptoms/Side effects	? Question ☆ To do

Date	Notes/Questions/To do's/Symptoms/Side effects	? Question ☆ To do

Date	Notes/Questions/To do's/Symptoms/Side effects	? Question ☆ To do

Date	Notes/Questions/To do's/Symptoms/Side effects	? Question ☆ To do

Date	Notes/Questions/To do's/Symptoms/Side effects	? Question ☆ To do

Date	Notes/Questions/To do's/Symptoms/Side effects	? Question ☆ To do

Date	Notes/Questions/To do's/Symptoms/Side effects	? Question ☆ To do

Date	Notes/Questions/To do's/Symptoms/Side effects	? Question ☆ To do

Date	Notes/Questions/To do's/Symptoms/Side effects	? Question ☆ To do

Date	Notes/Questions/To do's/Symptoms/Side effects	? Question ☆ To do

Date	Notes/Questions/To do's/Symptoms/Side effects	? Question ☆ To do

Date	Notes/Questions/To do's/Symptoms/Side effects	? Question ☆ To do

Date	Notes/Questions/To do's/Symptoms/Side effects	? Question ☆ To do

Date	Notes/Questions/To do's/Symptoms/Side effects	? Question ☆ To do

Date	Notes/Questions/To do's/Symptoms/Side effects	? Question ☆ To do

Date	Notes/Questions/To do's/Symptoms/Side effects	? Question ☆ To do

Date	Notes/Questions/To do's/Symptoms/Side effects	? Question ☆ To do

Date	Notes/Questions/To do's/Symptoms/Side effects	? Question ☆ To do

Date	Notes/Questions/To do's/Symptoms/Side effects	? Question ☆ To do

Date	Notes/Questions/To do's/Symptoms/Side effects	? Question ☆ To do

Date	Notes/Questions/To do's/Symptoms/Side effects	? Question ☆ To do

Date	Notes/Questions/To do's/Symptoms/Side effects	? Question ☆ To do

Thank You, Thank You! Journal

Here is a place to keep track of well wishes, gifts, and kind gestures that you receive from friends and family. Keeping a record will mean that you will not miss anyone, if later on you choose to send out thank-you cards, make phone calls, or send e-mail messages of gratitude.

Sometimes it is the unexpected visit, or that special phone call that made your day...

There are many ways to say *thank you* to those who have helped you through the treatment and recovery process. One woman threw a thank-you party to celebrate her recovery and her good friends. Remember, too, friends and family will say that no thanks is necessary; they were glad for a chance to have helped in some way.

Who	What

Who	What

Who	What

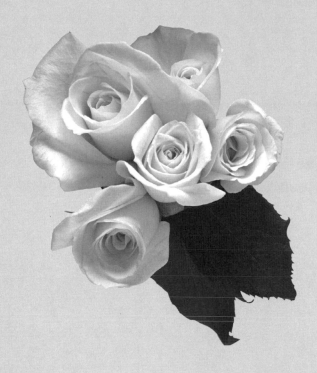

Record Keeping

MY MEDICAL HISTORY

BREAST CANCER TREATMENT HISTORY

MEDICATION LOG

MEDICAL AND LAB TESTS RECORD

INSURANCE INFORMATION AND MEDICAL EXPENSES

INSURANCE ISSUES AND HELP

MEDICAL BILLS AND EXPENSES TRACKER

Record Keeping

If you are seeing a doctor or specialist for the first time, you will be asked to provide information about your insurance coverage, health history, and your cancer treatment history. **You will be asked for this information over and over during the course of your treatment.**

To make it easier for you to provide your doctor with the best information on your initial visits, this book has convenient forms to help you gather the most often requested information.

○ Get copies of past medical records, including tests from the previous year. You can generally obtain these records at no charge, or ask your previous doctor to forward them to your new doctor.

○ Gather your immediate family's health history. Ask your blood relatives—parents, siblings, grandparents, aunts, uncles, and children—if they have had the conditions listed on the next page.

○ For each initial doctor or specialist visit, bring this book with you or bring copies of:

Your medical history and your family history on the next page.

Your health insurance information on page 123.

Your medications log and recent laboratory results on page 117.

Your cancer treatment medical history on page 112.

> **You will be asked for your medical history again and again.**

My Medical History

Name _____ Age _____

Date of Birth _____ Height _____ Weight _____

Emergency Contact _____

Phone _____ Relationship _____

Primary Physician _____ Phone _____

Surgeon _____ Phone _____

Radiation Oncologist _____ Phone _____

Other Doctor _____ Phone_____

Recent Breast Cancer Diagnosis _____ Date of Diagnosis _____

Known Allergies _____

_____

_____

_____

_____

Tobacco: Currently smoke? _____ Quit smoking in the year _____

I have _____ alcoholic drinks per week.   How often do you exercise? _____ hours per week.

IMMUNIZATIONS: Please list dates of last immunizations.

Hepatitis A ____/___   Pneumovax (pneumonia) ____/___

Hepatitis B ____/___   Meningitis ____/___

Influenza (flu shot) ____/___   Tetanus (Td) ____/___

HEALTH SCREENING TESTS:

Colonoscopy Date ____/___ Abnormal? Yes/No

Pap Smear Date ____/___ Abnormal? Yes/No

Bone Density (osteporosis) Date ____/___ Abnormal? Yes/No

PERSONAL HISTORY: Have you ever have had any of the following? Check (✔) all that apply:

___ Heart Disease   ___ Other Disease _____

___ Asthma /Lung Disease   ___ High Cholesterol

___ High Blood Pressure   ___ Thyroid Problem

___ Diabetes   ___ Kidney Disease

                                                    ___ Other Cancer _____

SURGICAL HISTORY: Please list all prior operations and dates:

_____

_____

_____

_____

_____

_____

_____

_____

_____

_____

_____

_____

_____

_____

_____

_____

_____

FAMILY HISTORY: Please indicate if family members (parent, sibling, grandparent, aunt, or uncle) have experienced the following:

Alcoholism _____ High Cholesterol _____

Cancer (specify type) _____

_____

_____

_____

_____

_____

_____

High Blood Pressure _____ Heart Disease _____ Stroke _____

Depression/Suicide _____ Bleeding or Clotting Disorder _____

Genetic Disorders _____ Asthma/COPD _____

Diabetes _____ Other: _____

Breast Cancer Treatment History

Name _____ Date of Birth _____

Date of Diagnosis of Breast Cancer _____

SURGERY

Type _____

Hospital _____

Surgeon _____ Phone _____

Date and Length of Stay _____

Type _____

Hospital _____

Surgeon _____ Phone _____

Date and Length of Stay _____

CHEMOTHERAPY

Oncologist _____ Phone _____

Total Number of Treatments _____

Date of First Treatment _____ Date of Last Treatment _____

Medications and Side Effects _____

_____

_____

_____

RADIATION THERAPY

Treatment _____ Total Number of Treatments _____

Date of First Treatment _____ Date of Last Treatment _____

OTHER THERAPY

Treatment Type _____

Treatment Dates _____

Side Effects _____

_____

_____

_____

Medication Log

Use this form to record all of the medicines that you are currently taking, including vitamins, over-the-counter medications, and supplements. Share this list with all your doctors.

Pharmacy Telephone Number _____

Known Allergies _____

Medication name:			What it is for:		Side effects experienced:
Refill no:					
Ordered by:	Dose:	How often:	Date started:	Date ended:	

Medication name:			What it is for:		Side effects experienced:
Refill no:					
Ordered by:	Dose:	How often:	Date started:	Date ended:	

Medication name:			What it is for:		Side effects experienced:
Refill no:					
Ordered by:	Dose:	How often:	Date started:	Date ended:	

Medication name:			What it is for:		Side effects experienced:
Refill no:					
Ordered by:	Dose:	How often:	Date started:	Date ended:	

Medication name:			What it is for:		Side effects experienced:
Refill no:					
Ordered by:	Dose:	How often:	Date started:	Date ended:	

Medication name:			What it is for:		Side effects experienced:
Refill no:					
Ordered by:	Dose:	How often:	Date started:	Date ended:	

Medication name:			What it is for:		Side effects experienced:
Refill no:					
Ordered by:	Dose:	How often:	Date started:	Date ended:	

Medication name:			What it is for:		Side effects experienced:
Refill no:					
Ordered by:	Dose:	How often:	Date started:	Date ended:	

Medication Log

Use this form to record all of the medicines that you are currently taking, including vitamins, over-the-counter medications, and supplements. Share this list with all your doctors.

Pharmacy Telephone Number _____

Known Allergies _____

Medication name:			What it is for:		Side effects experienced:
Refill no:					
Ordered by:	Dose:	How often:	Date started:	Date ended:	

Medication name:			What it is for:		Side effects experienced:
Refill no:					
Ordered by:	Dose:	How often:	Date started:	Date ended:	

Medication name:			What it is for:		Side effects experienced:
Refill no:					
Ordered by:	Dose:	How often:	Date started:	Date ended:	

Medication name:			What it is for:		Side effects experienced:
Refill no:					
Ordered by:	Dose:	How often:	Date started:	Date ended:	

Medication name:			What it is for:		Side effects experienced:
Refill no:					
Ordered by:	Dose:	How often:	Date started:	Date ended:	

Medication name:			What it is for:		Side effects experienced:
Refill no:					
Ordered by:	Dose:	How often:	Date started:	Date ended:	

Medication name:			What it is for:		Side effects experienced:
Refill no:					
Ordered by:	Dose:	How often:	Date started:	Date ended:	

Medication name:			What it is for:		Side effects experienced:
Refill no:					
Ordered by:	Dose:	How often:	Date started:	Date ended:	

Medication Log

Use this form to record all of the medicines that you are currently taking, including vitamins, over-the-counter medications, and supplements. Share this list with all your doctors.

Pharmacy Telephone Number _____

Known Allergies _____

Medication name: Refill no:			What it is for:		Side effects experienced:
Ordered by:	Dose:	How often:	Date started:	Date ended:	

Medication name: Refill no:			What it is for:		Side effects experienced:
Ordered by:	Dose:	How often:	Date started:	Date ended:	

Medication name: Refill no:			What it is for:		Side effects experienced:
Ordered by:	Dose:	How often:	Date started:	Date ended:	

Medication name: Refill no:			What it is for:		Side effects experienced:
Ordered by:	Dose:	How often:	Date started:	Date ended:	

Medication name: Refill no:			What it is for:		Side effects experienced:
Ordered by:	Dose:	How often:	Date started:	Date ended:	

Medication name: Refill no:			What it is for:		Side effects experienced:
Ordered by:	Dose:	How often:	Date started:	Date ended:	

Medication name: Refill no:			What it is for:		Side effects experienced:
Ordered by:	Dose:	How often:	Date started:	Date ended:	

Medication name: Refill no:			What it is for:		Side effects experienced:
Ordered by:	Dose:	How often:	Date started:	Date ended:	

Medication Log

Use this form to record all of the medicines that you are currently taking, including vitamins, over-the-counter medications, and supplements. Share this list with all your doctors.

Pharmacy Telephone Number _____

Known Allergies _____

Medication name:			What it is for:		Side effects experienced:
Refill no:					
Ordered by:	Dose:	How often:	Date started:	Date ended:	

Medication name:			What it is for:		Side effects experienced:
Refill no:					
Ordered by:	Dose:	How often:	Date started:	Date ended:	

Medication name:			What it is for:		Side effects experienced:
Refill no:					
Ordered by:	Dose:	How often:	Date started:	Date ended:	

Medication name:			What it is for:		Side effects experienced:
Refill no:					
Ordered by:	Dose:	How often:	Date started:	Date ended:	

Medication name:			What it is for:		Side effects experienced:
Refill no:					
Ordered by:	Dose:	How often:	Date started:	Date ended:	

Medication name:			What it is for:		Side effects experienced:
Refill no:					
Ordered by:	Dose:	How often:	Date started:	Date ended:	

Medication name:			What it is for:		Side effects experienced:
Refill no:					
Ordered by:	Dose:	How often:	Date started:	Date ended:	

Medication name:			What it is for:		Side effects experienced:
Refill no:					
Ordered by:	Dose:	How often:	Date started:	Date ended:	

Medical and Lab Tests Record

Request copies of all test results as the information develops. DO NOT WAIT. Test results are owned by you. Copies generated as they occur do not create a burden for the medical staff. Having this information for reference in the future will be valuable.

Lab Tests Explained. Here are two good resources for helping you understand the numbers behind your lab tests.

www.Labtestsonline.org is a brilliant Web site designed to help you better understand the many clinical lab tests that are part of routine care, as well as diagnosis and treatment of a broad range of conditions and diseases. You can search for information by condition, such as breast cancer, or by a specific test.

In addition, the Leukemia & Lymphoma Society has produced a booklet *Understanding Lab and Imaging Tests*. To order your free copy, call 800-955-4572 or go to *www.lls.org*.

It is also very helpful to keep a summary log of your test results for blood work, mammograms, x-rays, and bone scans during and after your treatments.

Date	Test	Result	Any Action Needed?
9/2/11	*CBC (Complete Blood Count)*	*WBC = 2500 low range*	*Retest – 1 week*

Date	Test	Result	Any Action Needed?

Date	Test	Result	Any Action Needed?

Date	Test	Result	Any Action Needed?

Insurance Information and Medical Expenses

For many, health insurance coverage and billing can become stressful because of confusion about benefits coverage, procedures, and the huge volume of medical bills and statements. With the treatment of breast cancer, you may need services from a number of different medical practices depending upon your situation—gynecologist, oncologist, radiologists, anesthesiologist, as well as imaging centers, testing laboratories, hospital centers, and pharmacies. So you can see how this could quickly amount to a lot of paperwork.

To help ease the stress, try to stay ahead of the situation and take the following steps:

1. Enter your insurance information on page **123**. Make copies of this information to bring with you to your appointments. As with your medical history and medication log, you will be asked for this information again and again. If you bring *The Breast Cancer Companion* to your appointments, you will have a handy record for the billing staff.

2. Set up a couple of file folders at home:

    Bills and Statements

    Explanation of Claims Reimbursement

3. Use the **Medical Bills and Expenses Tracker** on page **133** to keep track of who has been paid and how much, as well as insurance reimbursements.

4. Call your health care insurers and review your benefits and their procedures. Questions will arise about what your health insurance company does and does not cover, as well as how to get approval for reimbursement for specialists' visits, medications, and procedures. Early on, you can reduce your anxiety and potential stressful situations by calling the customer service telephone number of your insurance provider to discuss your diagnosis and treatment plan. You may choose to have a family member or friend make this call for you and act as your advocate on insurance matters. Use the question guide on page **124** for this conversation with the health insurance company.

5. If you need help resolving an insurance issue, see the resources on page **126** for groups who may be able to provide you with support.

When your primary care physician refers you to other health care providers, always get a referral. Ask for a prescription before you buy a wig during chemotherapy or a postmastectomy prosthesis. If your health policy requires you to have a referral before you see a massage therapist for lymphedema or to consult with a bone marrow specialist, be sure you have a referral before you go to your appointment. This referral can make the difference between a claim that is paid and a claim that is denied.

What if I Do Not Have Insurance?

First, ask if your hospital has a social worker that you can speak to about your situation. Social workers may know of hospital funds or other resources, such as free clinics, that can provide financial aid and/or free services.

Next, contact the following organizations for assistance:

- Call your local Social Services Department to see if you are eligible for Medicaid or other programs for those with low income. To find your local office, go to *www.benefits.gov* or call 1-800-FED-INFO (or 1-800-333-4636).

- The National Breast Cancer Coalition (NBCC) provides a guide for finding free or low-cost services (see NBCC's excellent guide on their Web site in the section: ACCESS: Finding Affordable Care [*www.stopbreastcancer.org*]).

- National Cancer Institute's Cancer Information Service maintains a list of national organizations that offer financial assistance to people with cancer and their families. Call 1-800-4-CANCER (1-800-422-6237) (*www.cancer.gov*).

- Call your local Public Health Department to find out about local health care programs available in your area.

Prescriptions

The Partnership for Prescription Assistance brings together America's pharmaceutical companies, doctors, other health care providers, patient advocacy organizations, and community groups to help qualifying patients who lack prescription coverage get the medicines they need through the public or private program that is right for them. Qualified patients will get their medications free or nearly free (*www.pparx.org*).

Health Insurer Information

PRIMARY HEALTH CARE INSURER:

Name of Insurance Company _____

Subscriber Number _____ Group Number _____

Type of Policy (HMO, PPO) _____

Name of Insured _____

Phone: Claims and Authorizations _____

Phone: Customer Service (Information) _____

E-mail or Web Site _____

Address for Correspondence _____

_____

Case Manager (if assigned) _____

PRIMARY HEALTH CARE INSURER:

Name of Insurance Company _____

Subscriber Number _____ Group Number _____

Type of Policy (HMO, PPO) _____

Name of Insured _____

Phone: Claims and Authorizations _____

Phone: Customer Service (Information) _____

E-mail or Web Site _____

Address for Correspondence _____

Case Manager (if assigned) _____

TIPS

- Keep a copy of your benefits descriptions for easy reference.
- Always get a referral before you go to see other specialists and therapists.
- Ask for a prescription before you buy a wig or prosthesis.
- Save a record of all correspondence with your insurance company.
- Keep a copy of claim forms and copies of bills.
- Use the Medical Bills and Expenses Tracker to keep up with the insurance claims filed and paid.
- Write down in the insurance phone log on page 127 the date and name of each person that you speak to.
- Consider choosing a case manager to act on your behalf for all insurance matters (discussed later).

A Guide for Your Conversation With Your Health Insurance Company

Case Manager

Will this insurance company provide me with a case manager to help me understand my benefits and coordinate my plan coverage for the treatment of breast cancer?

_____

Primary Physician

Are visits to the primary physician covered? _____

Is there a limit on how many visits? _____

How much is my co-pay fee for each visit? _____

Other Doctors

Does the plan cover the fees of specialists, such as an oncologist, surgical oncologist, and radiation oncologist? _____

Do I need a referral before I see these specialists? _____

What is the procedure for getting a referral? _____

Do these doctors have to be part of a specific insurance carrier network?

_____

What if the doctor whom I want to see is not part of my insurance carrier network?

_____

Second Opinions

As you decide on your course of treatment, it is recommended that you obtain additional opinions about your diagnosis and treatment plan.

Does my plan cover second opinions? _____

Surgery

May I have my surgery at any clinic or hospital, or only those facilities approved by your insurance company?

_____

I am planning to have the surgery as an outpatient. Does my plan cover the cost of a home health nurse to come to my home postsurgery? How many visits are allowed?

_____

Chemotherapy

Does my plan cover chemotherapy treatments? _____

What if I plan to participate in a clinical trial? _____

In the event that I lose my hair during chemotherapy treatments, does my plan cover the cost of a wig? _____

What is the procedure to obtain reimbursement?

_____

_____

Note: If your health plan does not cover the cost of a wig, check with the American Cancer Society for assistance. See **Resources**, page **144**.

Radiation Therapy

Does my plan cover radiation treatments? _____

May I receive your radiation treatment at any clinic or hospital, or only those facilities approved by your insurance company? _____

Reconstruction or Prosthesis

What is the procedure for obtaining reimbursement for a prosthesis?

_____

What is the procedure for obtaining coverage for breast reconstruction surgery?

_____

What is the extent of coverage for each section of treatment?

_____

Note: If you have had a mastectomy or expect to have one, you may be entitled to special rights under the Women's Health and Cancer Rights Act (WHCRA) of 1998 regarding your group health plan reconstructive surgery and other postmastectomy benefits.

_____

Medications

Does my insurance plan pay for my medications? _____

Are there limitations? _____

Is there a co-pay fee for prescriptions? _____ How much? _____

Is there a prescription plan to reduce costs? _____

Insurance Issues and Help

Getting reimbursed for medical expenses can quickly become complicated, especially when there are a number of doctors and various treatments, tests, prescriptions, home care, and, in some cases, clinical trials. It can also be very stressful, particularly if claims and services are denied or reimbursed at a reduced level.

This is the time to get help from family and friends with filling out the paperwork and dealing with the insurance company. As mentioned before, find out if your insurance company will provide you with a case manager who will help you coordinate your treatment options and the payments of your medical expenses.

Your Health Insurance Rights

The Georgetown University Health Policy Institute has written *A Consumer Guide for Getting and Keeping Health Insurance* for each state. These consumer guides are available at *www.healthinsuranceinfo.net* and will be updated periodically as changes in federal and state policy warrant.

Do You Need an Advocate?

The Patient Advocate Foundation is a national nonprofit organization that helps patients with the specific issues they are facing with their insurer, employer, and/or creditor regarding insurance, job retention, and/or debt crisis matters relative to their diagnosis of life threatening or debilitating diseases (*www.patientadvocate.org*).

CancerCare is a national nonprofit organization that provides free, professional support services to anyone affected by cancer. CancerCare may be able to provide help resolving insurance issues (*www.CancerCare.org*).

Health Insurance Phone Log

Keep track of every conversation with your insurance company.

Date	Name	Comments

Date	Name	Comments

Date	Name	Comments

Date	Name	Comments

Date	Name	Comments

Date	Name	Comments

Medical Bills and Expenses Tracker

Keeping track of medical expenses can be confusing and stressful. Use the following aids to help you be organized.

Keep a copy of your benefits descriptions for easy reference.

Save a record of all correspondence with your insurance company.

Keep a copy of claim forms and copies of bills. Use the **Medical Bills and Expenses Tracker** on the next page to keep up with the insurance claims that have been filed and those that have been paid.

Taxes

Medical expenses above and beyond what is paid by your insurance company can be substantial. If your medical and dental expenses exceed 7.5% of your adjusted gross income, you may deduct your medical expenses from your federal taxes.

In general, the following expenses (less any amounts reimbursed by your insurance company) are deductible:

- All medical expenses
- Out-of-pocket travel expenses to medical care (24 cents/mile in 2009)
- Prescription medications
- Medical supplies and equipment
- Insurance premiums (the amount that you contribute)
- Mental illness costs

Store all of your receipts. Refer to the Internal Revenue Service (IRS) if you have questions.

Web site: *www.irs.gov/taxtopics/tc502.html*

or *www.irs.gov*

Phone: 1-800-829-1040

Medical Bills and Expenses Tracker

DATE OF BILL	MEDICAL OFFICE	INVOICE NUMBER	DESCRIPTION OF SERVICES	AMOUNT BILLED	DATE OF CLAIM SENT	AMOUNT PAID INSURANCE	BALANCE DUE

Medical Bills and Expenses Tracker

DATE OF BILL	MEDICAL OFFICE	INVOICE NUMBER	DESCRIPTION OF SERVICES	AMOUNT BILLED	DATE OF CLAIM SENT	AMOUNT PAID INSURANCE	BALANCE DUE

Medical Bills and Expenses Tracker

DATE OF BILL	MEDICAL OFFICE	INVOICE NUMBER	DESCRIPTION OF SERVICES	AMOUNT BILLED	DATE OF CLAIM SENT	AMOUNT PAID INSURANCE	BALANCE DUE

Medical Bills and Expenses Tracker

DATE OF BILL	MEDICAL OFFICE	INVOICE NUMBER	DESCRIPTION OF SERVICES	AMOUNT BILLED	DATE OF CLAIM SENT	AMOUNT PAID INSURANCE	BALANCE DUE

Medical Bills and Expenses Tracker

DATE OF BILL	MEDICAL OFFICE	INVOICE NUMBER	DESCRIPTION OF SERVICES	AMOUNT BILLED	DATE OF CLAIM SENT	AMOUNT PAID INSURANCE	BALANCE DUE

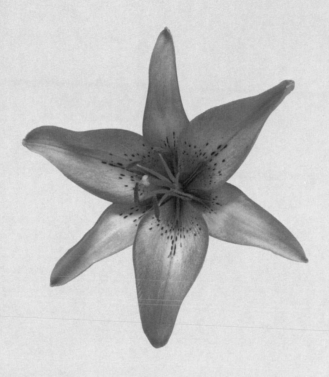

Resources

INFORMATION

Learn as Much as You Can

MAGAZINES AND BOOKS

Magazines

Books

INFORMATION AND SUPPORT ORGANIZATIONS

SHOPPING!

Resources

Information

Learn as Much as You Can

The more you know, the better you can work with your doctors to manage your treatment. When diagnosed with breast cancer, you will become aware of the vast amount of information and news available about breast cancer from various sources. As you learn more, share your information with your doctors. They will be able to explain how this information relates to your situation.

In addition to learning about treatment options, you may want to seek out information about the "lifestyle therapies" of nutrition, exercise, and stress reduction. These are areas where you can be especially proactive to learn and do things that will help you be as strong and healthy as possible as you go through your treatments and recovery.

Information, news, and support:

○ **Books and Brochures**—There are many books available about treating and living with breast cancer. Amazon.com lists more than 3,000 titles relating to breast cancer. Ask your support team for their recommendations. At a minimum, consider getting a copy of *Dr. Susan Love's Breast Book* (discussed later), which is considered "the bible for women with breast cancer" (*The New York Times*) as a reliable reference guide for at home.

○ **Information and Support Organizations**—There are many excellent and informative organizations for women with breast cancer that provide research and support. Always ensure that the information and news have been reviewed by medical experts.

○ **Newspapers and Magazine Articles**—Daily newspapers and magazines can be good sources of information for ongoing tips for living well and good health. Clip out articles for yourself or to share with your doctor and support groups. It is important to confirm that this information is accurate and from reputable sources! Your health care team can help you do this.

○ **Nightly News and Investigative Broadcasts**—The broadcast media can also be a good source of the latest information about breast cancer research and treatments. Listen carefully for the names of doctors and medical facilities during a broadcast in the event that you would like to follow up on the reports.

Magazines and Books
Magazines
LIVE**STRONG** *Quarterly*

*LIVE**STRONG** Quarterly* is a new print, online, and print-on-demand magazine. The publication bolsters our efforts to make cancer a global priority through compelling profiles of advocates, survivors, and supporters in the fight against cancer. Each issue contains articles on health, fitness, and wellness, as well as resources and information about preventing, treating, and raising cancer awareness. The focus is to build an engaging community to take meaningful action on cancer issues (www.livestrongmagazine.com).

Coping With Cancer

Coping With Cancer magazine is written by and for the cancer community. A wide variety of professionals share their knowledge and experience in easy-to-read, relevant articles, and patients, caregivers, and survivors share their strategies for coping. Also included are the latest news, FDA updates, resource lists, and interviews with celebrity cancer survivors.

CURE

CURE is a quarterly magazine with an annual resource guide and special issue that combines the science and humanity of cancer for those who have to deal with it on a daily basis. *CURE* provides scientific information in easy-to-understand language, with equally understandable illustrations.

"tlc" (Tender Loving Care)

"tlc" is an American Cancer Society publication, a combination of magazine and catalog. This "magalog" provides special products and information for women newly diagnosed with breast cancer and for breast cancer survivors. *"tlc"* can be viewed online, or a print copy can be ordered at no cost to you in the following ways:

- ○ Visit the *tlc* Web site at: *www.tlcdirect.org*
- ○ To request a print copy: call 1-800-850-9445, or write to: tlc, PO Box 395, Louisiana, MO 63353-0395

HEAL: Living Well After Cancer

HEAL: Living Well After Cancer is for cancer survivors starting from the day treatment ends and continuing for the rest of their lives. Topics covered by *HEAL* include cancer's aftereffects, optimal nutrition and fitness, survivor stories, and more.

Books

Breast Cancer: Clear and Simple from the American Cancer Society. This complete and easy-to-understand book subtitled *All Your Questions Answered* will be a welcome resource in the first weeks after your diagnosis (*www.cancer.org*).

Dr. Susan Love's Breast Book by Susan M. Love, MD, with Karen Lindsey and Marcia Williams, is considered the bible of breast cancer and the essential guide to understanding your medical pathology.

The Breast Cancer Survival Manual (fourth edition) by John Link, MD, is a step-by-step guide for the woman with newly diagnosed cancer. It empowers the reader to navigate through the second opinion process and to make confident treatment plan decisions.

The Breast Cancer Reconstruction Handbook (second edition) by Kathy Steligo is highly recommended by breast cancer patients as a blueprint of the reconstruction process. This book explains the benefits and limitations of each reconstructive technique, and what to expect each step of the way: before your surgery, in the hospital, during recovery, and life beyond reconstruction.

Crazy Sexy Cancer Tips by Kris Carr is an uplifting and sassy look at coping with a cancer diagnosis. Includes a fabulous nutrition guide and recipes, as well as lifestyle choices for supporting your immune system.

Living Through Breast Cancer by Carolyn M. Kaelin MD, MPH, with Francesca Coltrera. Dr. Kaelin is a breast cancer surgeon and director of the Comprehensive Breast Health Center and Brigham and Women's Hospital in Boston. Diagnosed with breast cancer in 2003, she had three lumpectomies, a mastectomy, chemotherapy, and reconstructive surgery. She shares valuable information from the unique perspectives as expert and survivor.

Ramy Gafni's Cancer Beauty Therapy: The Ultimate Guide to Looking and Feeling Great While Living With Cancer by Ramy Gafni, a professional makeup artist to the stars, who offers practical solutions and step-by-step instructions for managing the dermatologic "damage" done by cancer treatments.

Yoga and Breast Cancer: A Journey to Health and Healing by Ingrid Kollack, RN, and Isabell Utz, MD. More than simply an exercise book, *Yoga and Breast Cancer* is a deeply soothing form of moving meditation and physical activity that is a safe way to rebuild strength, stamina, and flexibility both during and following cancer treatments. It will support women during the critical phases of their disease, as well as during times of secondary prevention and rehabilitation.

Information and Support Organizations

American Cancer Society

The American Cancer Society is a nationwide, community-based, volunteer health organization dedicated to eliminating cancer as a major health problem by preventing cancer, saving lives, and diminishing suffering from cancer, through research, education, advocacy, and service (www.cancer.org or 1-800-ACS-2345).

Provides information, education, and support services including:

> ***Reach to Recovery*** *offers visits—face-to-face visits or by phone—with volunteers who give support and up-to-date information, including literature for spouses, children, friends, and other loved ones. Volunteers can also, when appropriate, provide breast cancer patients with a temporary breast form and information on types of permanent prostheses, as well as lists of where those items are available within a patient's community.*

> ***"tlc" (Tender Loving Care)*** *is a "magalog" (magazine/catalog) that combines helpful articles and information with products for women coping with cancer or any cancer treatment that causes hair loss. Products include wigs, hairpieces, breast forms, prostheses, bras, hats, turbans, swimwear, and helpful accessories at the lowest possible prices.*

> ***Look Good . . . Feel Better*** *program is a community-based, free, national service that teaches female cancer patients beauty techniques to help restore their appearance and self-image during chemotherapy and radiation treatments.*

American Society of Clinical Oncology

The American Society of Clinical Oncology (ASCO) is the voice of the world's cancer physicians. ASCO has created an oncologist-approved Web site for patients, Cancer.Net, making it the most up-to-date and trusted resource for cancer information on the Internet (www.cancer.net/patient or 1-571 483-1300).

Breastcancer.org

Breastcancer.org is a nonprofit organization dedicated to providing the most reliable, complete, and up-to-date information about breast cancer. Their mission is to help women and their loved ones make sense of the complex medical and personal information about breast cancer, so they can make the best decisions for their lives (www.breastcancer.org).

Breast Cancer Network of Strength (Formerly Known as Y-ME National Breast Cancer Organization)

The mission of the Breast Cancer Network of Strength is to ensure, through information, empowerment, and peer support, that no one faces breast cancer alone (www. networkofstrength.org).

Breastlink.com

*This Web site provides a terrific explanation about the importance of second opinion, in addition to other valuable resources. The Breastlink Medical Group, founded by Dr. John Link, implements a team-based approach at its breast cancer centers in southern California. Dr. Link is the author of **The Breast Cancer Survival Manual** (mentioned earlier) (www.breastlink.com, or 310-791-6610).*

Cancer Consultants

An award winning Web site that provides access to the most current information about the prevention, screening, treatment, and overall management of cancer (www.patientcancerconsultants.com).

ChemoCare.Com

ChemoCare.com is an extensive Web site that provides the latest about chemotherapy to patients and their families, caregivers, and friends. Detailed information about chemotherapy drugs, strategies to manage side effects, complementary therapy, and more is available (www.chemocare.com).

ECaP Exceptional Cancer Patients

Dr. Bernie Siegel's site provides tools, information, and resources based on the science of mind-body healing (www.ecap-online.org or 814-337-8192).

Fertile Hope

Fertile Hope is dedicated to providing reproductive information, support, and hope to cancer patients and survivors whose medical treatments present the risk of infertility (www.fertilehope.org or 888-994-HOPE [888-994-4673]).

Force

Force is dedicated to providing support and information resources for women at risk of hereditary breast cancer based on family history or BRCA genetic status (www.facingourrisk.org).

HER2 Support Group

Information and support for women whose breast cancer is HER2 positive (www.her2support.org or 760-602-9178).

Inflammatory Breast Cancer Research Foundation

The Inflammatory Breast Cancer Research Foundation is dedicated to researching the cause of inflammatory breast cancer (IBC) (www.ibcresearch.org or 877-STOP-IBC [877-786-7422]).

Living Beyond Breast Cancer

Information on breast cancer treatment, testing, side effects, clinical trials, and treatment options (www.lbbc.org, 1-888-753-LBBC [1-888-753-5222], or 610-645-4567).

Necessities Bag

Ask your surgeon or surgery nurse about obtaining a Necessities Bag before your mastectomy surgery. The Necessities Bag is a reusable tote filled with bandages and essentials for wound care, hygiene, and personal comfort. This invaluable tote is distributed for free by medical professionals. It was created by Maureen Lutz whose personal experience with cancer gave her a perspective on how she should have prepared for her needs in the hospital and afterward at home (www.necessitiesbag.org).

The National Comprehensive Cancer Network

The National Comprehensive Cancer Network (NCCN) is an alliance of 21 of the world's leading cancer centers, working together to develop treatment guidelines for most cancers, and dedicated to research that improves the quality, effectiveness, and efficiency of cancer care. NCCN offers a number of programs to help you and your family make informed decisions about your health (www.nccn.com).

The National Lymphedema Network

Provides extensive education and guidance to lymphedema patients (www.lymphnet.org).

SHARE: Self-Help for Women With Breast or Ovarian Cancer

SHARE has nationwide hotlines staffed by trained and knowledgeable volunteers who are cancer survivors (www.sharecancersupport.org or 866-891-2392).

Shop Well With You

Shop Well With You (SWY) is a not-for-profit organization and body-image resource for women surviving cancer, their caregivers, and health care providers. Through its Web site, SWY focuses on helping women improve their self-image and quality of life (www.shopwellwithyou.org).

Susan G. Komen Breast Cancer Foundation

The Komen Breast Cancer Foundation is the world's largest and most progressive grassroots network of breast cancer survivors. The foundation's mission is to eradicate breast cancer as a life-threatening disease by advancing research, education, screening, and treatment. It involves millions of participants in fundraisers, such as the Komen Run for the Cure in communities across the country (www.Komen.org).

Young Survival Coalition

Dedicated to the concerns and issues that are unique to young women with breast cancer (www.youngsurvival.org).

Shopping!

Hospital Clothing Designed for Breast Cancer Patients

Shop Well With You

This is not a shopping site but should be your first stop. The *Shop Well With You* (SWY) site has a fabulous and comprehensive directory for clothing and accessories for women surviving cancer. "SWY focuses on helping women improve their self-image and quality of life" (*www.shopwellwithyou.org*).

Healing Threads

Elegant, soft, and cozy hospital jackets and pants with Velcro enclosures to allow easy access for treatments (*www.spirited-sisters.com* or *1-877-647-3900*).

Assistwear Garments

Provides a line of hospital garments designed to be worn at the hospital and during recuperation. These garments made of comfortable, easy care, and fashionable fabric are designed for wear immediately after any surgery requiring drainage bulbs, including breast augmentation, breast reduction, cancer surgery, and abdominoplasty (*www.assistwear.com*).

Still You Fashions

Supplies an exceptional line of comfortable and attractive prosthetic alternatives for women who are in all stages of postoperative breast cancer (*www.stillyoufashions.com*).

TheBreastCareSite.com

This site is sponsored by Amoena, the worldwide leader in postmastectomy products, and carries a line of intimate apparel, swimwear, breast forms, symmetry shapers, and postoperative products. In addition, this site focuses on providing breast cancer survivors with information about everything from postsurgery options and products, to information about insurance and intimacy issues (*www.TheBreastCareSite.com*).

Glossary

A

ablative therapy: treatment that removes or destroys the function of an organ.

adenocarcinoma: cancer that starts in glandular tissue, such as in ducts or lobules of the breast.

adenoid cystic carcinoma or adenocystic carcinoma: a rare type of breast cancer that has both glandular and cylinder-like features when looked at under the microscope.

adenoma: a non-cancer growth that starts in the glandular tissue.

adjuvant therapy: treatment used in addition to the main treatment. The term can refer to hormone therapy, chemotherapy, or radiation therapy added after surgery to increase the chances of curing the disease or keeping it in check.

alopecia: hair loss, which may include eyebrows, eyelashes, and pubic hair. This can happen as a result of chemotherapy. In most people, the hair grows back after treatment ends.

alternative therapy: use of an unproven therapy instead of standard (proven) therapy. Some alternative therapies have dangerous or even life-threatening side effects that may not be well known. With others, the main danger is that the patient may lose the chance to benefit from standard therapy.

anesthesia: the drug-induced loss of feeling or sensation. General anesthesia causes loss of consciousness (makes you go to sleep). Local or regional anesthesia numbs only a certain area of the body.

angiogenesis: the formation of new blood vessels. Some cancer treatments work by preventing the tumor from forming blood vessels.

antibiotic: a drug used to kill organisms (germs) that cause disease. Antibiotics may be made naturally by living organisms, or they may be man-made in the lab. Antibiotics may be used to treat or prevent infections.

antiemetic: a drug that prevents or relieves nausea and vomiting.

antiestrogen: a drug that blocks the effects of estrogen on breast tumors. Antiestrogens are used to treat breast cancers that depend on estrogen for growth.

areola: normal darkened area of skin surrounding the nipple of the breast.

aromatase inhibitors: drugs that keep the adrenal glands from making estrogens. They are used to treat hormone-sensitive breast cancer in postmenopausal women. Anastrozole (Arimidex), letrozole (Femara), and exemestane (Aromasin) are some examples.

aspiration: the process of drawing out fluid or cells by suction from a body cavity.

atypical: not usual; abnormal. Refers to the appearance of cells under the microscope. The presence of these cells is sometimes described as **atypia**.

axilla: the armpit.

axillary lymph node dissection or axillary dissection: surgical removal of the lymph nodes from the armpit (axillary nodes). They are looked at under a microscope to see if they contain cancer.

B

Benign: not cancer; not malignant. Benign breast problems can be referred to as fibroadenomas or fibrocystic changes.

bilateral: affecting on both sides of the body; for example, bilateral breast cancer is cancer in both breasts.

biologic response modifiers: an agent that boosts normal immune response to fight against cancer.

biopsy: removing a sample of tissue for microscopic examination to see whether cancer cells are present.

brain scan: an imaging test used to find anything not normal in the brain. This test can be done in an outpatient clinic. It is painless, except for the needle stick when a radioactive substance is injected into an arm vein. The images taken will show where radioactivity builds up, which is a sign that the area may be cancer.

BRCA1, BRCA2: a gene containing inherited alterations which places a woman at much greater risk of developing breast and/or ovarian cancer, compared with women who do not have the alteration.

BRCAPRO: a tool used to help health professionals estimate a woman's breast cancer risk.

breast augmentation: surgery to increase the size of the breast.

breast cancer: cancer that starts in the breast.

breast conserving therapy or breast conservation therapy: surgery to remove a breast cancer and a small amount of normal tissue around the cancer, without removing any other part of the breast. This method is also called *lumpectomy*, *segmental excision*, *limited breast surgery*, or *tylectomy*.

breast implant: a liquid or solid material used to increase breast size or to restore the shape of the breast after mastectomy.

breast reconstruction: surgery done to rebuild the breast after mastectomy. Choices include the use of artificial implants or tissue from the women's own body.

breast self-exam (BSE): a method of checking one's own breasts for changes. The goal with BSE is to know what your breast tissue feels and looks like, and to be able to report any breast changes to a doctor or nurse right away.

breast specialist: a doctor or nurse who has a dedicated interest in breast health. He or she will have specialized knowledge in this area.

C

CAT scan or CT scan: Can detect extremely small tumors that may not be seen on an X-ray.

calcifications: tiny calcium deposits within the breast, either alone or in clusters, usually found by mammography. They are a sign of change within the breast that may need to be followed by more mammograms or by a biopsy. Calcifications may be caused by benign breast conditions or by breast cancer.

chemo brain: the mental cloudiness people with cancer sometimes notice after chemotherapy. Despite the name, its exact cause is uncertain.

chemotherapy: treatment with drugs to kill cancer cells.

D

digital mammography: a method of storing an x-ray image of the breast as a computer image rather than on the usual x-ray film. Digital mammography can be combined with **computer-aided detection (CAD)**, a process in which the radiologist uses a computer program to help interpret the mammogram. This method requires less radiation than traditional mammography.

dose-dense chemotherapy: giving the usual doses of chemo closer together (every 2 weeks) rather than the every-3-week schedule.

doubling time: the time it takes for a cell or a cancer to divide and double itself. The doubling time of breast cancer cells depends on many things, such as the type of tumor, the resistance of the individual's body, and the location in which it tries to grow.

duct: a narrow tubular passage that carries a liquid from a gland.

ductal carcinoma in situ (DCIS): cancer that starts in cells in the milk passages (ducts) and does not break through the duct walls into the nearby tissue. This is a highly curable form of breast cancer that is treated with surgery or surgery plus radiation therapy.

ductogram: a test in which a fine plastic tube goes into the nipple and injects a contrast dye that outlines the shape of the duct. X-rays are then taken to see if there is a mass.

E

edema: buildup of fluid in the tissues, causing swelling. Edema of the arm can occur after radiation or surgery, such as radical mastectomy or axillary dissection of lymph nodes.

endocrine glands: glands that release hormones into the bloodstream.

endocrine therapy: the use of hormones to treat a disease or condition.

estrogen: a female sex hormone produced by the ovaries and in smaller amounts by the adrenal glands. In women, levels of estrogen and other hormones work together to regulate the development of secondary sex characteristics, including breasts; regulate the monthly cycle of menstruation; and prepare the body for fertilization and reproduction. In breast cancer, estrogen may promote the growth of cancer cells.

estrogen receptor assay: a lab test done on a sample of the cancer to see if estrogen receptors are present. Growth of normal breast cells and some breast cancers are stimulated by estrogen. Estrogen receptors are molecules that function as a cell's "welcome mat" for estrogen circulating in the blood. Breast cancer cells without these receptors (called **estrogen receptor–negative** or **ER-negative**) are unlikely to respond to hormonal therapy. Cancers with estrogen receptors (**ER-positive**) are likely to respond to hormonal therapy.

estrogen replacement therapy: the use of estrogen from sources other than the body. Estrogen may be given after a woman's body no longer makes its own supply. This type of hormone therapy is often used to relieve symptoms of menopause in women who no longer have a uterus.

external beam radiation therapy (EBRT): radiation that is focused from a source outside the body on the area affected by the cancer. It is much like getting a diagnostic x-ray, but for a longer time and at a higher dose.

accelerated breast irradiation: use of a slightly larger than usual dose of radiation each day, so that the course of radiation can be completed in a shorter time.

intraoperative radiation: a single large dose of radiation given in the operating room following a lumpectomy. This is a type of accelerated partial breast radiation, in that it does not treat the whole breast but only the affected area.

F

fluorescent in situ hybridization (FISH): a test used to detect HER2/neu protein in breast cancer biopsy samples. This protein is a marker of a more aggressive cancer that may benefit from new drugs.

frozen section: a very thin slice of tissue that has been quick-frozen and then looked at under a microscope. This method is done during an operation because it gives a quick diagnosis. The diagnosis is confirmed within a few days by a more detailed study called a *permanent section*.

G

gene: a basic unit of heredity that contains information on hereditary characteristics such as hair color, eye color, or height, as well as tendency to have certain diseases. Women who have BRCA1 or BRCA2 gene mutations (defects) have an inherited (genetic) tendency to develop breast cancer.

genetic counseling: the process of counseling people who may have inherited a gene that makes them more likely to develop cancer.

genetic counselor: a specially trained health professional who educates and supports people as they consider genetic testing.

genetic testing: tests done to see if a person has inherited certain gene changes known to increase breast cancer risk. Such testing is not recommended for everyone, but rather for those with specific types of family history.

glands: secretory organs that produce and release substances used in other parts of the body.

grade: the grade of a cancer reflects how different its cells look compared with normal cells under the microscope. There are several grading systems for breast cancer, but all divide cancers into those with the greatest abnormality (grade 3 or poorly differentiated), the least abnormality (grade 1 or well differentiated), and those with intermediate features (grade 2 or moderately differentiated). Grading is done by the pathologist who looks at the tumor tissue under a microscope. Along with the cancer's stage, the grade is used to help determine the best treatment options. A cancer's **nuclear grade** is based on features of the central part of its cells, the nucleus. The **histologic grade** is based on features of individual cells, as well as how the cells are arranged together.

H

HER2 gene: (Human epidermal growth factor receptor 2), a gene that is stimulated to produce an excess of protein.

high risk: when the chance of developing cancer is greater than that normally seen in the general population. People may be at high risk because of a family history of breast cancer.

hormone: a chemical substance released into the body by the endocrine glands, such as the thyroid, adrenals, or ovaries. Hormones travel through the bloodstream and set in motion various body functions.

hormone receptor: a protein located in or on a cell that binds a hormone. Tumors can be tested for hormone receptors to see if they can be treated with hormones or hormone-like substances.

hormone receptor assay: a test to see if a breast tumor is likely to be affected by hormones and if it can be treated with hormones.

hormone replacement therapy or HRT: the use of estrogen and progesterone from an outside source after the body has stopped making its own supply because of natural or induced menopause. This type of hormone therapy is often given to relieve symptoms of menopause in women who still have a uterus.

hormone therapy: treatment with hormones, with drugs that interfere with hormone production or hormone action, or the surgical removal of hormone-producing glands to kill cancer cells or slow their growth.

I

in situ: in place; localized and confined to one area. A very early stage of cancer.

inflammatory breast cancer: a type of invasive breast cancer, which spreads to lymphatic vessels in the skin covering the breast. The skin of the affected breast is red, feels warm, and may thicken to look and feel like an orange peel. A lump is not necessarily present.

invasive cancer: cancer that has spread beyond the layer of cells where it started and into nearby tissues.

invasive ductal carcinoma: a cancer that starts in the milk passages (ducts) of the breast and then breaks through the duct wall and spreads into the fatty tissue of the breast. It can spread elsewhere in the breast, as well as to other parts of the body through the bloodstream and lymphatic system. Invasive ductal carcinoma is the most common type of breast cancer, accounting for about 80% of breast malignancies.

invasive lobular carcinoma: a cancer that starts in the milk-producing glands (lobules) of the breast and then breaks through the lobule walls to spread into nearby fatty tissue. About 10% of invasive breast cancers are invasive lobular carcinomas. It is often difficult to detect by physical examination or even by mammography.

L

latissimus dorsi flap procedure: a method of breast reconstruction in which skin, fat and muscle is taken from the person's abdomen, back or buttock.

lobular carcinoma in situ (LCIS): although not a true cancer, LCIS is classified as a type of noninvasive cancer. It develops within the milk-producing glands (lobules) of the breast and does not break through the wall of the lobules. Researchers think that LCIS cells almost never progress to invasive lobular cancer. But having LCIS puts a woman at a higher risk of developing an invasive breast cancer later. For this reason, it is important for women with LCIS to have an annual mammogram and clinical breast exam.

localized breast cancer: cancer starts in the breast and is confined to the breast.

lumpectomy: surgery to remove the breast tumor and a small amount of the normal tissue around it.

lymph nodes: small bean-shaped collections of immune system tissue, such as lymphocytes, found along lymphatic vessels. They remove cell waste, germs, and other harmful substances from lymph. They help fight infections and also have a role in fighting cancer.

lymphedema: swelling caused by a collection of excess fluid in the arms. This may happen after the lymph nodes and vessels are surgically removed or are injured by radiation, and it can happen many years after treatment.

M

mammogram, mammography: an x-ray of the breast; a way to find breast cancers that cannot be felt. Mammograms are done with a special type of x-ray machine that is used only for this purpose. A mammogram can show a developing breast tumor before it is large enough to be felt by a woman or even by a highly skilled health care professional.

mammoplasty: any plastic surgery to reconstruct the breast or to change the shape, size, or position of the breast. Reduction mammoplasty reduces the size of the breast. Augmentation mammoplasty enlarges a woman's breast.

margin: the edge of the cancerous tissue or lump removed during surgery. A negative surgical margin is a sign that no cancer was left behind. A positive surgical margin means that cancer cells are found at the outer edge of the removed sample.

mastectomy: surgery to remove all or part of the breast and sometimes other tissue. There are different types of mastectomy:

> *Modified radical mastectomy* removes the breast, skin, nipple, areola, and most of the axillary lymph nodes on the same side, leaving the chest muscles intact.

> *Partial mastectomy* removes less than the whole breast, taking only the part of the breast in which the cancer occurs and a margin of healthy breast tissue surrounding the tumor.

> *Prophylactic mastectomy* is a mastectomy done before any evidence of cancer can be found. This procedure is sometimes recommended for women at very high risk of breast cancer.

> *Quadrantectomy* is a partial mastectomy in which the quarter of the breast that contains a tumor is removed.

> *Segmental mastectomy* is a partial mastectomy.

> *Simple mastectomy* or *total mastectomy* removes only the breast and areola.

> *Skin-sparing mastectomy* leaves as much of the breast skin as possible to improve the way the reconstructed breast looks.

> *Subcutaneous mastectomy* is surgery to remove internal breast tissue. The nipple and skin are left intact.

metastasis: the movement of cancer cells from one organ to another body part.

N

needle aspiration: a type of needle biopsy done to remove fluid from a cyst or cells from a tumor.

needle biopsy: removal of fluid, cells, or tissue with a needle to be looked at under a microscope. There are two types: **fine needle aspiration** (also called FNA or needle aspiration)and core biopsy. FNA uses a thin needle and syringe to pierce the skin and draw up fluid or small tissue fragments from a cyst or tumor. A **core needle biopsy** uses a thicker needle to remove a piece of tissue from a tumor.

needle localization: a procedure used to guide a surgical breast biopsy when the lump is hard to find or when there are areas that look suspicious on the mammogram but there is not a distinct lump. A thin needle is placed into the breast. X-rays are then used to guide the needle to the suspicious area. The surgeon then uses the path of the needle as a guide to find the abnormal area to be removed.

neoadjuvant therapy: systemic therapy, such as chemotherapy or hormone therapy, given before surgery. This can shrink some breast cancers, so that surgical removal can be done with a less-extensive operation than would otherwise be needed.

O

osteoporosis: thinning of bone tissue, resulting in less bone mass and weaker bones. Osteoporosis can cause pain, deformity, and broken bones. This condition is common among postmenopausal women and can be caused by many factors.

P

pathologist: a doctor who specializes in diagnosing changes in a tissue removed during the time of a biopsy or operation.

positron emission tomography (PET): a type of imaging test that places radioactive sugar in a vein. A special camera then makes detailed pictures of the places where the radioactive sugar collects signally a possible cancer.

progesterone: a female sex hormone released by the ovaries during every menstrual cycle to prepare the uterus for pregnancy and the breasts for milk production.

progesterone receptor assay: a lab test done on a breast cancer specimen that shows whether the cancer depends on progesterone for growth. Progesterone and estrogen receptor tests provide information to help in deciding the best cancer treatment for the patient.

R

radiation: high-energy ionizing particles that are used for x-rays and, in higher doses, for cancer treatment.

radiation therapy: treatment with ionizing radiation and particles to kill cancer cells. The radiation may come from outside of the body, and may be given in different ways. Radiation may also come from radioactive materials placed directly in the tumor. Radiation therapy may be used to reduce the size of a cancer before surgery, to destroy any remaining cancer cells after surgery, or in some cases, as the main treatment. In advanced cancer cases, it may also be used as palliative treatment.

raloxifene: a drug that blocks the effects of estrogen on breast tissue. The brand name is Evista.

S

selective estrogen receptor modulator (SERM): a man-made estrogen-like substance that possesses some, but not all, of the actions of estrogen.

sentinel lymph node biopsy (SLNB): A blue dye and/or a radioactive tracer is injected into the tumor site at the time of surgery, and the first (sentinel) node that picks up the dye is removed and biopsied. If the node is cancer free, fewer nodes are removed. Also known as *sentinel node biopsy*.

stereotactic needle biopsy: a method of needle biopsy that is useful in some cases where there are calcifications or a mass that can be seen on mammogram but cannot be felt. A computer maps the location of the mass to guide the placement of the needle. When this type of biopsy is done with a larger needle, it may be called a **stereotactic core needle biopsy**.

surgical biopsy: a method of biopsy in which all or part of a lump is removed by a surgeon for diagnosis.

survivorship: Quality of life issues that permeate every aspect of life after diagnosis of cancer.

systemic therapy: treatment that reaches and affects cells throughout the body.

T

tamoxifen: a drug that blocks the effects of estrogen on many organs, such as the breast. Brand name is Nolvadex. Tamoxifen can be used to treat or reduce the risk of breast cancer recurrence. It is also used as a preventative medication in high-risk women.

transverse rectus abdominus muscle (TRAM) flap procedure: a method of breast reconstruction in which tissue from the lower abdominal wall, which gets its blood supply from the rectus abdominus muscle, is used. The tissue from this area is moved up to the chest to create a breast mound and usually does not require an implant. Moving muscle and tissue from the lower abdomen to the chest results in flattening of the lower abdomen (a "tummy tuck").

triple-negative breast cancer: breast cancer that does not have estrogen receptors, progesterone receptors, or human epidermal growth factor receptor 2 (HER2).

tumor: a new growth forming an abnormal mass with unknown origin.

Index